Psychodynamic Psychiatry

Editor

THOMAS N. FRANKLIN

PSYCHIATRIC CLINICS OF NORTH AMERICA

www.psych.theclinics.com

Consulting Editor
HARSH K. TRIVEDI

June 2018 • Volume 41 • Number 2

ELSEVIER

1600 John F. Kennedy Boulevard • Suite 1800 • Philadelphia, Pennsylvania, 19103-2899

http://www.theclinics.com

PSYCHIATRIC CLINICS OF NORTH AMERICA Volume 41, Number 2
June 2018 ISSN 0193-953X, ISBN-13: 978-0-323-61058-2

Editor: Lauren Boyle
Developmental Editor: Kristen Helm

Psychiatric Clinics of North America (ISSN 0193-953X) is published quarterly by Elsevier Inc., 360 Park Avenue South, New York, NY 10010-1710. Months of issue are March, June, September, and December. Business and Editorial Offices: 1600 John F. Kennedy Blvd., Suite 1800, Philadelphia, PA 19103-2899. Periodicals postage paid at New York, NY and additional mailing offices. Subscription prices are $321.00 per year (US individuals), $666.00 per year (US institutions), $100.00 per year (US students/residents), $391.00 per year (Canadian individuals), $460.00 per year (international individuals), $838.00 per year (Canadian & international institutions), and $220.00 per year (Canadian & international students/residents). Foreign air speed delivery is included in all *Clinics*' subscription prices. All prices are subject to change without notice. **POSTMASTER:** Send address changes to *Psychiatric Clinics of North America*, Elsevier Health Sciences Division, Subscription Customer Service, 3251 Riverport Lane, Maryland Heights, MO 63043. **Customer Service: 1-800-654-2452 (US). From outside the United States, call 1-314-447-8871. Fax: 1-314-447-8029. E-mail: journalscustomerservice-usa@elsevier.com (for print support)** and **journalsonline support-usa@elsevier.com (for online support)**.

Reprints. For copies of 100 or more, of articles in this publication, please contact the Commercial Reprints Department, Elsevier Inc., 360 Park Avenue South, New York, New York 10010-1710. Tel.: 212-633-3874, Fax: 212-633-3820, E-mail: reprints@elsevier.com.

Psychiatric Clinics of North America is covered in *MEDLINE/PubMed (Index Medicus)*, *Current Contents/Social and Behavioral Sciences, Social Science Citation Index, Embase/Excerpta Medica,* and PsycINFO.

Contributors

CONSULTING EDITOR

HARSH K. TRIVEDI, MD, MBA
President and CEO, Sheppard Pratt Health System, Baltimore, Maryland, USA

EDITOR

THOMAS N. FRANKLIN, MD
Medical Director, The Retreat at Sheppard Pratt, Sheppard Pratt Health System, Baltimore, Maryland, USA

AUTHORS

AIDA SYARINAZ A. ADLAN, MBBS, MPM
Senior Lecturer and Consultant Psychiatrist, Department of Psychological Medicine, University of Malaya, Kuala Lumpur, Malaysia

CÉSAR A. ALFONSO, MD
Associate Professor, Department of Psychiatry, Columbia University Medical Center, New York, New York, USA; Visiting Professor, Department of Psychiatry, National University of Malaysia, Kuala Lumpur, Malaysia

FREDRIC N. BUSCH, MD
Clinical Professor of Psychiatry, Weill Cornell Medical College, Faculty, Columbia University Center for Psychoanalytic Training and Research, New York, New York, USA

JENNIFER I. DOWNEY, MD
Clinical Professor of Psychiatry, Columbia University, New York, New York, USA

KATERINA DUCHONOVA, MD
Psychiatrist, Military University Hospital Prague, Prague, Czech Republic

SYLVIA DETRI ELVIRA, MD
Psychiatrist, Department of Psychiatry, Universitas Indonesia, Jakarta, DKI Jakarta, Indonesia

RICHARD C. FRIEDMAN, MD
Clinical Professor of Psychiatry, Weill Cornell Medical College, New York, New York, USA

GLEN O. GABBARD, MD
Clinical Professor of Psychiatry, Baylor College of Medicine, Training and Supervising Analyst, Center for Psychoanalytic Studies, Houston, Texas, USA

RICHARD G. HERSH, MD
Columbia University Medical Center, New York, New York, USA

BRIAN JOHNSON, MD
Member, Boston Psychoanalytic Society & Institute, Newton Centre, Massachusetts, USA; Professor of Psychiatry and Anesthesia, Department of Psychiatry, Director of Addiction Medicine, State University of New York (SUNY) Upstate Medical University, Syracuse, New York, USA

RASMON KALAYASIRI, MD
Associate Professor, Department of Psychiatry, Chulalongkorn University, Bangkok, Thailand

KATHERINE G. KENNEDY, MD
Assistant Clinical Professor, Department of Psychiatry, Yale Medical School, New Haven, Connecticut, USA

SUSAN G. LAZAR, MD
Clinical Professor of Psychiatry, George Washington University School of Medicine & Health Sciences, Supervising and Training Analyst, Washington Psychoanalytic Institute, Washington, DC, USA; Uniformed Services University of the Health Sciences, Bethesda, Maryland, USA

PETRIN REDAYANI LUKMAN, MD, MMedEd
Psychiatrist, Department of Psychiatry, Universitas Indonesia, Jakarta Pusat, DKI Jakarta, Indonesia

MARCO CHRISTIAN MICHAEL, MD, BMedSc
Research Assistant, Department of Psychiatry, Universitas Indonesia, Jakarta, DKI Jakarta, Indonesia

BARBARA L. MILROD, MD
Professor of Psychiatry, Weill Cornell Medical College, Faculty, The New York Psychoanalytic Institute, Columbia University Center for Psychoanalytic Training and Research, New York, New York, USA

DAVID MINTZ, MD
Staff Psychiatrist, Director of Psychodynamic Psychopharmacology Initiative, Austen Riggs Center, Stockbridge, Massachusetts, USA

MAHDIEH MOINALGHORABAEI, MD
Assistant Professor of Psychiatry, Tehran University of Medical Sciences, Tehran, Iran

ERIC M. PLAKUN, MD
Associate Medical Director, Director of Biopsychosocial Advocacy, Austen Riggs Center, Stockbridge, Massachusetts, USA

MOHAMMAD SAN'ATI, MD
Assistant Professor of Psychiatry, Tehran University of Medical Sciences, Tehran, Iran

JONATHAN SHEDLER, PhD
Clinical Associate Professor, Department of Psychiatry, University of Colorado School of Medicine, Denver, Colorado, USA

BARRY L. STERN, PhD
Columbia University College of Physicians and Surgeons, Columbia University Center for Psychoanalytic Training and Research, New York, New York, USA

TIMOTHY B. SULLIVAN, MD
Associate Professor, Department of Psychiatry, Hofstra Northwell School of Medicine, Staten Island, New York, USA

ELIZABETH WEINBERG, MD
Staff Psychiatrist, Austen Riggs Center, Stockbridge, Massachusetts, USA

FRANK YEOMANS, MD, PhD
NewYork Presbyterian Hospital, Weill Cornell Medical College, Cornell University, New York, New York, USA

MICHAEL YOUNG, MD, MS
Psychiatrist, Sheppard Pratt Health System Volunteer Faculty, University of Maryland/ Sheppard Pratt Psychiatry Residency Training Program, Towson, Maryland, USA

HAZLI ZAKARIA, MBBS
Psychiatrist, Department of Psychiatry, National University of Malaysia, Kuala Lumpur, Malaysia

Contents

Foreword: Psychodynamic Psychiatry **xiii**

Harsh K. Trivedi

Preface: Psychodynamic Psychiatry: Clinical, Practical, Patient Centered, and Evidence-Based **xv**

Thomas N. Franklin

On the Birth of Psychodynamic Psychiatry **177**

Richard C. Friedman, Jennifer I. Downey, and César A. Alfonso

Psychodynamic psychiatry emerged from psychoanalytic theory, but the influence of the latter has been only partial. Equally important are other disciplines outlined within this article. Modern psychodynamic publications and presentations should honor all of the foundational pillars of the field. In this way, the new area lends itself to biopsychosocial integrations that remain a challenge for all researchers and clinicians who seek to understand and treat patients with mental disorders.

Preserving the Person in Contemporary Psychiatry **183**

Glen O. Gabbard

Psychodynamic psychiatry is a way of thinking that places the person at the heart of diagnostic understanding and treatment. This emphasis on unique characteristics of an individual is at odds with much of contemporary psychiatric thought, which is geared to identifying a set of criteria designed to identify discrete diagnostic categories with biological underpinnings. This article addresses component parts of the person that are linked to psychodynamic constructs and lie at the heart of diagnostic understanding and treatment in psychodynamic psychiatry.

The Place for Psychodynamic Therapy and Obstacles to Its Provision **193**

Susan G. Lazar

Psychodynamic treatment provides benefits for patients with personality disorders, chronic depressive and anxiety disorders, and chronic complex disorders, and its intensity and duration have independent positive effects. Obstacles to its provision include a bias privileging brief treatments, especially cognitive behavior therapy, seen as a gold standard of treatment, despite difficulties with the design of, and ability to generalize from, its supporting research and the diagnostic nosology of the illnesses studied. Another obstacle lies in insurance company protocols that violate the mandate for mental health parity and focus on conserving insurers' costs rather than the provision of optimum treatment to patients.

The Psychodynamic Treatment of Borderline Personality Disorder: An Introduction to Transference-Focused Psychotherapy 207

Barry L. Stern and Frank Yeomans

The authors describe the application of a twice-weekly exploratory psychotherapy, transference-focused psychotherapy (TFP), to patients with borderline personality disorder. The article describes the pathology of internal object relations that provides a framework for understanding borderline personality and how TFP establishes a treatment framework to address such pathology and set the stage for working at the level of internal psychological structure. An outline of the assessment and treatment protocol is described along with a case example to illustrate the same.

A Psychodynamic Approach for the General Psychiatrist: Using Transference-Focused Psychotherapy Principles in Acute Care Settings 225

Richard G. Hersh

Transference-focused psychotherapy (TFP) is one of the empirically validated treatments for patients with borderline personality disorder. TFP has roots in psychoanalytically informed psychotherapy, although important elements of the treatment have been adapted and refined for patients with significant personality disorder pathology. TFP's assessment process is informed by the structural interview, an approach that synthesizes standard DSM-5 nosology with the psychodynamic concept of the personality organization. TFP principles can be integrated into practice in general psychiatry settings in the care of patients with primary or co-occurring personality disorder pathology.

Psychodynamic Psychiatry, the Biopsychosocial Model, and the Difficult Patient 237

Eric M. Plakun

This article defines psychodynamic psychiatry as the intersection between general psychiatry and psychoanalysis as a theory of mind. Psychodynamic psychiatry is built on a biopsychosocial model for understanding and treating mental disorders. Currently, a narrower biomedical model is in ascendancy, but it has not lived up to its promise and is not supported by emerging science as robustly as is the biopsychosocial model. The "difficult patient" emerges in part from the limits of our treatment models and treatment methods. Concepts such as projective identification and enactment help us to understand our own contributions to our experience of a patient as difficult.

Treatment-Resistant Depression: The Importance of Identifying and Treating Co-occurring Personality Disorders 249

Michael Young

Treatment-resistant depression (TRD) presents a significant burden to individuals and society, and comprehensive, individualized approaches are needed to address this complex clinical situation. Diagnostic reevaluation is indicated in cases of TRD to determine the numerous factors that could be playing a role in the treatment resistance. Factors to assess during the diagnostic reevaluation are discussed, including assessment for personality disorders, which are common contributors to treatment resistance and are often not adequately addressed. Two case studies are presented to illustrate the importance of addressing underlying personality disorders in the setting of chronic depression and TRD.

The Overall Diagnosis: Psychodynamic Psychiatry, 6-Minute Psychotherapy, and Patient-Centered Care **263**

Elizabeth Weinberg and David Mintz

Optimal patient care in psychiatry necessitates attention to the treatment relationship and to the patient's experience as an individual. The growth of patient-centered medicine has led to an increased appreciation of the importance of the biopsychosocial formulation, the personhood of both the patient and the physician, the autonomy and authority of the patient, and the therapeutic alliance. Patient-centered medicine, developed by the seminal psychoanalytic theorist Michael Balint, has its roots in psychodynamic concepts. A psychodynamic approach to psychopharmacology improves psychiatric prescribing and guides the psychiatrist in providing brief, limited psychotherapy, similar to that which Balint recommended in primary care practice.

Trauma-Focused Psychodynamic Psychotherapy **277**

Fredric N. Busch and Barbara L. Milrod

The authors describe a psychodynamic psychotherapeutic approach to posttraumatic stress disorder (PTSD), trauma-focused psychodynamic psychotherapy. This psychotherapy addresses disruptions in narrative coherence and affective dysregulation by exploring the psychological meanings of symptoms and their relation to traumatic events. The therapist works to identify intrapsychic conflicts, intense negative affects, and defense mechanisms related to the PTSD syndrome using a psychodynamic formulation that provides a framework for intervention. The transference provides a forum for patients to address feelings of mistrust, difficulties with authority, fears of abuse, angry and guilty feelings, and fantasies.

Advocacy for Psychodynamic Psychotherapy: Challenges and Benefits **289**

Katherine G. Kennedy

Psychodynamic psychotherapy, also called psychodynamic therapy (PDT), is an effective mental health treatment that is currently under siege on several fronts. It is at risk of being effectively excluded from the future of American health care. Psychiatrists need to learn how to advocate for a future mental health care delivery system that assures their patients have access to PDT. This article examines the stigma against both psychiatrists and PDT, identifies some of the challenges to advocacy that psychiatrists face, and offers an approach to developing the necessary skills that psychiatrists need to advocate effectively for PDT.

Innovative Educational Initiatives to Train Psychodynamic Psychiatrists in Underserved Areas of the World 305

César A. Alfonso, Marco Christian Michael, Sylvia Detri Elvira, Hazli Zakaria, Rasmon Kalayasiri, Aida Syarinaz A. Adlan, Mahdieh Moinalghorabaei, Petrin Redayani Lukman, Mohammad San'ati, Katerina Duchonova, and Timothy B. Sullivan

Psychodynamic psychiatry remains a challenging subject to teach in underserved areas, where enthusiasm to learn is substantial. Besides logistical and psychiatric workforce shortcomings, sensible cultural adaptations to make psychodynamic psychiatry relevant outside of high-income countries require creative effort. Innovative pedagogic methods that include carefully crafted mentoring and incorporate videoconferencing in combination with site visits can be implemented through international collaborations. Emphasis on mentoring is essential to adequately train future psychodynamic psychotherapy supervisors. Examples of World Psychiatric Association initiatives in countries such as Indonesia, Iran, Malaysia, and Thailand are presented as possible models to emulate elsewhere.

Where Is the Evidence for "Evidence-Based" Therapy? 319

Jonathan Shedler

The term evidence-based therapy is a de facto code word for manualized therapy, most often brief cognitive behavior therapy and its variants. It is widely asserted that "evidence-based" therapy is scientifically proven, superior to other forms of psychotherapy, and the gold standard of care. Research findings do not support such assertions. Research on evidence-based therapies demonstrates that they are weak treatments. They have not shown superiority to other forms of psychotherapy, few patients get well, and treatment benefits do not last. Questionable research practices create a distorted picture of the actual benefits of these therapies.

Engineering Neurobiological Systems: Addiction 331

Brian Johnson

Neurobiological engineering is the process of making models of brain function and psychoanalytic psychology as these interact in a social environment to hide complexity while remaining true to science. One-fourth of Americans are killed by drugs. The engineering model described is applied to psychodynamic therapy of addicted patients. It helps us understand why addiction is ubiquitous, hostile, malicious, and intractable. Drugs take over the will by changing the ventral tegmental dopaminergic SEEKING system.

PSYCHIATRIC CLINICS OF NORTH AMERICA

FORTHCOMING ISSUES

September 2018
Neuromodulation
Scott T. Aaronson and Noah S. Philip, *Editors*

December 2018
Borderline Personality Disorder
Frank Yeomans and Kenneth N. Levy, *Editors*

RECENT ISSUES

March 2018
Geriatric Psychiatry
Dan G. Blazer and Susan K. Schultz, *Editors*

December 2017
Cognitive Behavioral Therapy for Anxiety and Depression
Stefan G. Hofmann and Jasper J.A. Smits, *Editors*

RELATED INTEREST

Primary Care: Clinics in Office Practice, June 2016 (Vol. 43, No. 2)
Psychiatric Care in Primary Care Practice
Janet R. Albers, *Editor*
Available at: http://www.primarycare.theclinics.com/

Foreword
Psychodynamic Psychiatry

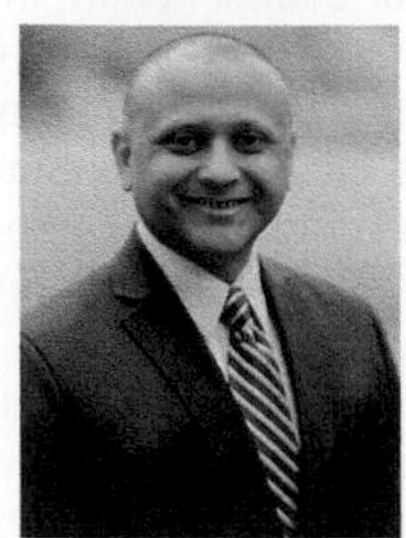

Harsh K. Trivedi, MD, MBA
Consulting Editor

The journey of a thousand miles begins with a single step.

—Lao Tzu

Welcome! It is a privilege to serve as the first Consulting Editor of the *Psychiatric Clinics of North America*. I began this journey ten years ago, when I became Consulting Editor for the *Child and Adolescent Psychiatric Clinics of North America* in 2008. While much was accomplished with that series, the vibrancy of a scientific publication is based on academic curiosity and continual intellectual nourishment. As is customary for many academic journals, I felt that it was important to create a self-imposed "term limit." Such a change in leadership breathes new life and new ideas and maintains relevancy of the series. I am thankful for the talented and dedicated publishers at Elsevier with whom I have worked: Sarah Barth, Joanne Husovski, and Lauren Boyle. The *Child and Adolescent Psychiatric Clinics of North America* continues to flourish, and I wish continued success to its new Consulting Editor, Dr Todd Peters.

The opportunity to become the inaugural Consulting Editor of the *Psychiatric Clinics of North America* intertwines with a recent professional transition. In July of 2016, I became the President and CEO of Sheppard Pratt Health System (SPHS). Sheppard Pratt is the largest private, nonprofit provider of mental health, substance use, special education, and social support services in the country. Since its founding in 1853, SPHS has been an innovator in the fields of research and best practice implementation, with a focus on improving the quality of mental health care on a global level. As a nationwide resource, it has been consistently ranked as a top national psychiatric hospital by US News & World Report for the past 27 years. The breadth and depth of high-quality clinical services across the entire continuum of psychiatric care are a natural fit for the array of topics that this series covers. The focus on advancing care and propelling our field also aligns well with this series. As such, I am humbled to be given the opportunity to serve as the inaugural editor of the *Psychiatric Clinics of North America*. It is

Psychiatr Clin N Am 41 (2018) xiii–xiv
https://doi.org/10.1016/j.psc.2018.03.002

my sincere hope that we create content that inspires and educates you. I am excited to work alongside the editorial team to bring new and stimulating topics: to remain current, to remain relevant, and to continue lifelong learning.

This first issue is aptly titled, "Psychodynamic Psychiatry." It highlights the importance of Psychodynamic Psychiatry in twenty-first century medicine. In this age of technology, we refocus on how important relationships are to our overall health. In a world where people often speak with their digital assistants, such as "Siri" or "Alexa," we find that the relationship between care provider and patient is crucial to determining health outcomes across medicine. It is only by getting to know a patient and understanding the interconnection between their mind, brain, and social environment that we can promote the self-reflection and self-awareness that is integral to long-term recovery.

I thank Dr Thomas N. Franklin for his vision and leadership in crafting a very special issue. With the aid of a superb lineup of leaders in the field, he has crafted an issue that showcases the best of psychodynamic psychiatry. The issue illustrates the psychodynamic approach for so many of the disorders we treat, including borderline personality disorder, treatment-resistant depression, and posttraumatic stress disorder. It also presents psychodynamic psychiatry in the context of manualized therapies and poses thought-provoking questions about the place of each in current psychiatric care.

Welcome! I hope you enjoy this issue and look forward to a great lineup of future issues, of which we have already begun working.

Harsh K. Trivedi, MD, MBA
Sheppard Pratt Health System
6501 North Charles Street
Baltimore, MD 21204, USA

E-mail address:
htrivedi@sheppardpratt.org

Preface
Psychodynamic Psychiatry: Clinical, Practical, Patient Centered, and Evidence-Based

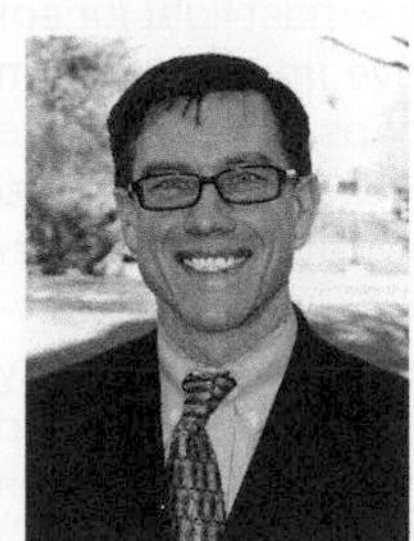

Thomas N. Franklin, MD
Editor

Welcome to the *Psychiatric Clinics of North America* issue on Psychodynamic Psychiatry. After reading this collection of articles, I think you will agree that psychodynamic psychiatry is an example of what twenty-first century medicine is aspiring to be: patient centered, evidence-based,[1,2] and concerned with the root causes of suffering and disability rather than simply treating symptoms as they arise.

Psychodynamic psychiatry approaches the patient as a human being rather than simply as a malfunctioning machine. If an ill person can be thought of as a pilot flying a plane, biomedical psychiatry's focus is simply on the smooth functioning of the aircraft. The psychodynamic psychiatrist is concerned not just with the engines and airframe but also with the pilot. She understands that the way the aircraft and pilot coexist and the feedback they give each other are critical in how the plane flies. She knows that the weather the plane is flying in affects its performance. The mind, brain, and the social environment cannot be approached in isolation if one wants the most effective alleviation of suffering and disability.

Interestingly, as psychiatry has followed pharmaceutical companies' oversimplified narrarative about the causes and best treatments of psychiatric illnesses, other medical specialties have discovered what psychodynamic psychiatrists have always known, that the *relationship* between treater and patient is critical to determining health outcomes of all kinds.[3] Indeed, loneliness itself is being recognized as one of the most important predictors of ill health.[4] The practitioners of psychodynamic psychiatry are some of the world experts in treating the underlying causes of social isolation through their deep and longstanding interest in helping people understand how their minds actually work in relation to other people. The psychodynamic psychiatrist uses the special relationship that exists between doctor and patient to fundamentally change how

Psychiatr Clin N Am 41 (2018) xv–xvi
https://doi.org/10.1016/j.psc.2018.03.001
0193-953X/18/© 2018 Published by Elsevier Inc.

people see themselves, the world, and their place in it. This may be through psychotherapy or in shorter encounters in the hospital or clinic.

The twenty-first century psychodynamic psychiatrist is practical and flexible in their approach to improving people's lives, becoming hyperfocused on neither biomedical symptom management nor endless philosophizing without ever honing in on what is actually causing the patient difficulty. There is not a religious devotion to a theory of mind or an insecure retreat from the human being in the room by seeing their suffering as a purely neurological illness.

For psychiatry to have a generative future, we must have more to offer than a symptom-focused diagnosis followed by algorithm-based prescribing. We must fight for access to intensive treatment when indicated and refocus the narrative from short-term symptom management to long-term recovery. Psychodynamic psychiatry is the bridge to the future that will not just help people but also allow the profession to stay relevant as the masters of the central force in all of health care by utilizing the therapeutic relationship.

Thomas N. Franklin, MD
The Retreat at Sheppard Pratt
Sheppard Pratt Health System
6501 North Charles Street
Baltimore, MD 21204, USA

E-mail address:
tfranklin@sheppardpratt.org

REFERENCES

1. Shedler J. The efficacy of psychodynamic psychotherapy. Am Psychol 2010;65: 98–109.
2. Lazar S. The cost-effectiveness of psychotherapy for the major psychiatric diagnoses. Psychodyn Psychiatry 2014;42:423–58.
3. Birkhäuer J, Gaab J, Kossowsky J, et al. Trust in the health care professional and health outcome: a meta-analysis. PLoS One 2017;12(2):e0170988.
4. Valtorta NK, Kanaan M, Gilbody S, et al. Loneliness and social isolation as risk factors for coronary heart disease and stroke: systematic review and meta-analysis of longitudinal observational studies. Heart 2016;102(13):1009–16.

On the Birth of Psychodynamic Psychiatry

Richard C. Friedman, MD[a,*], Jennifer I. Downey, MD[b], César A. Alfonso, MD[c]

KEYWORDS

- Psychodynamic psychiatry • Psychoanalysis • Organized psychiatry
- Diagnostic and Statistical Manual of Mental Disorders II

KEY POINTS

- Before publication of Diagnostic and Statistical Manual of Mental Disorders III, the prevailing model of the mind in organized psychiatry was psychoanalytic.
- The psychoanalytic model of the mind used in organized psychiatry before 1980 did not support reliability of psychiatric diagnosis.
- The psychoanalytic model of the mind used in organized psychiatry before 1980 was not based on and did not facilitate systematic research.
- After 1980, when the Diagnostic and Statistical Manual of Mental Disorders III was organized, atheoretically and descriptively, psychoanalytic ideas were systematically eliminated from organized psychiatry.
- Selected psychoanalytic ideas remain useful in psychiatry.

Psychodynamic psychiatry, in our view, is an emerging new discipline equally anchored in psychoanalysis, academic psychology, sexology, and academic psychiatry. To understand the circumstances of its emergence, it is necessary to review the many meanings the term *psychoanalysis* has assumed and been given in technical and lay parlance over the years.

With the publication of Diagnostic and Statistical Manual of Mental Disorders (DSM) III in 1980, organized psychiatry in the United States chose to change its framework with respect to its foundational models and paradigms. Whereas the DSM-I[1] and DSM-II[2] were psychoanalytically oriented, no subsequent edition of the DSM has been. Instead, a descriptive, Kraepelinian approach was adopted and persists.

This new perspective went beyond specifying criteria for psychiatric diagnoses. It was based on outright rejection of a psychoanalytically informed model of health and disease.

Disclosure Statement: N/A.
[a] Department of Psychiatry, Cornell Medical College, 525 East 68th Street, New York City, NY 10065, USA; [b] Department of Psychiatry, Columbia University, 108 East 91st Street # 1A, New York City, NY 10128, USA; [c] Department of Psychiatry, Columbia University Medical Center, 262 Central Park West, Suite #1B, New York City, NY 10024, USA
* Corresponding author.
E-mail address: rcf2@cumc.columbia.edu

Psychiatr Clin N Am 41 (2018) 177–182
https://doi.org/10.1016/j.psc.2018.01.009
psych.theclinics.com

Soon to follow was expurgation of psychoanalytic ideas, concepts, and perspectives from organized psychiatry in the United States. Before the third edition of the DSM for example, most department chairs and training directors were psychoanalytically trained.[3]

Organized psychoanalysis and psychiatry enjoyed a close relationship. Psychoanalysts made important contributions to developmental psychology and psychosomatic medicine[4] and many other areas of psychiatry. Nonetheless, the cultures and histories of the 2 disciplines led to incompatibilities that we discuss below and ultimately to a rupture between the 2 fields.

After 1980, the scientific literature of the 2 fields diverged. Most psychiatric journals avoided psychoanalytic ideas entirely. In fact, as of 2012 when this editorial team took over directorship of the official journal of the American Academy of Psychodynamic Psychiatry and Psychoanalysis, *Psychodynamic Psychiatry* has been the only English-language psychiatric journal that includes psychoanalytic ideas, concepts, and observations as part of its core contents.[4]

Although we disagree with this relatively recent direction of American psychiatry, we feel it is helpful to understand how it came about. This is especially important given the emergence of psychodynamic psychiatry as a new discipline within the larger field of psychiatry.

HISTORICAL ISSUES

Freud began his professional career as an academic physician whose career path was blocked because he was Jewish.[5] Private practice was the way he could make a living—and he soon became a successful practitioner.

This accident of fate seems to have wed organized psychoanalysis as it subsequently evolved to a private practice paradigm, rather than an experimentally based, empirical frame of reference. As academic psychiatry grew along an empirically validated path, psychoanalytic psychology gradually but somewhat disdainfully moved away from traditional academic research.

This movement was not only because so many of the psychoanalytic patients were neurotic, unlike the predominately psychotic population treated by psychiatrists in the past. The movement also took place because of insistence by many psychoanalysts that consciousness was merely a layer of the mind that happened to be immediately accessible. Under conscious awareness, unconscious motives lurked, and these unconscious fears and desires were often different in their ultimate meanings than conscious recall indicated. For example, a person who allegedly loved another might unconsciously hate her. Given this ambiguity of meaning, it was difficult to assess the motivational significance of consciously experienced psychic material or its role in symptom formation. Much academic psychology, however, was based on quantification of consciously accessible thoughts, feelings, and memories.

This information notwithstanding, it ultimately became necessary for psychiatrists to demonstrate that they could make diagnoses in a valid and reliable manner. Their poor capacity to do this contributed to the diminished influence of psychoanalysis in psychiatry.[6]

IMPORTANT RELEVANT ISSUES CREATING CONFLICT BETWEEN THE 2 DISCIPLINES

Many other issues produced conflict between the 2 disciplines. Below are listed just a few:

1. Psychoanalytic ideas about psychopathology are based almost entirely on data obtained from patients in treatment. The field emerged without attention to the

need for controlled studies, which inevitably led to a biased perspective supported almost entirely by induction without validation.

2. Psychoanalytic ideas about behavior are largely based on data that are observational only. Freud's ideas emerged from his reflections on individual and social behavior that happened to catch his attention. This happenstance methodology seemed to have more in common with humanistic fields than science and medicine.
3. Freud's speculations, hypotheses, and (so-called) conclusions were often mutually contradictory over time. He changed his ideas in a manner similar to the way an artist, like Picasso for example, changed his style over time.[7]
4. Freud emphasized the central role of the Oedipus complex in the development of health and illness. This theory has never been validated or adequately supported by extra-analytic evidence.[8] Modern research especially illuminates the role of genetics and psychosocial trauma in the development of psychopathology.
5. Freud's emphasis on the centrality of childhood sexual fantasies, memories, and experience in the genesis of psychopathology was challenged by the emergence of knowledge about sexual differentiation of brain and behavior. Much adult sexuality is the result of prenatal hormonal influences, an area largely unknown to Freud.[9]
6. Psychoanalytic societies across the world tend to emphasize different aspects of behavior as being of central importance in health and illness. Lacan,[10] Jung,[11] Jung,[12] and Horney[13] all stress different dimensions of behavior as being of crucial importance for example.

ADDITIONAL IDEAS AND CONCEPTS ORIGINALLY POSED BY FREUD

In trying to characterize the central aspects of psychoanalysis Freud also emphasized the following:

- The fundamental rule of clinical psychoanalytic practice states that during each analytical session the patient should verbalize whatever comes to mind, no matter how apparently trivial or irrelevant or socially unacceptable. Nothing must be held back.
- This verbalization leads to the emergence of transference—the patient's original infantile conflicts become directed toward the analyst—a substitute object.
- As these processes are experienced and expressed, resistances inevitably occur. The patient disguises her narrative to make understanding her associations more difficult.
- Also, infantile and now unconscious conflicts are organized by the primary process—here Freud observed a cognitive difference between unconscious, infantile organization of mentation and usual adult thought.
- In primary process thinking, ideas are not posed in terms of abstract, cause-and-effect reasoning, but rather the phenomena of condensation, symbolization, and displacement of emphasis shape the material. Time and space limitations imposed on everyday reasoning are abandoned.[14]

The way these concepts and those outlined earlier are used in contemporary articles must be selective. For example, one would be hard put to understand the etiology of conversion reactions without alluding to Freud's original contributions about the influence of infantile unconscious conflicts on symptom formation.[15] In contrast, it is not possible to discuss modern theories of depression or psychosis without deep understanding of genetics and also trauma theory. This understanding contributed to the genesis of psychodynamic psychiatry—field that uses some psychoanalytic ideas but is different from psychoanalysis.

RELATIONSHIP BETWEEN PSYCHOANALYSIS AND PSYCHODYNAMIC PSYCHIATRY

Psychodynamic psychiatry (the discipline) emerged recently for many reasons, some of which are outside the scope of this article. In our view, this new field of knowledge is one of the foundational pillars of all modern psychiatry. As such, it is important not to conflate it with psychoanalysis.

For example, psychodynamic psychiatry is a branch of psychiatry, not an extension of psychoanalysis. As a branch of psychiatry, its role in assessment, coping, and diagnosis is fundamentally important. This is the case for its role in psychodynamically oriented psychotherapy as well. Sometimes the terms *psychodynamic psychotherapy* and *psychodynamic psychiatry* are mistakenly conflated. This should be avoided, however, because psychodynamic psychiatry, in our view, is a much more inclusive term, connoting all of psychological development and functioning in health and illness.

PSYCHODYNAMIC PSYCHIATRY REJECTS POSTMODERNISM

Psychoanalytic psychology is, for the most part benignly positive in its attitude toward postmodernism. The notion that all narrative modes are inherently equally valid fits well with the need of psychoanalytic societies throughout the world to cast a wide net and welcome in practitioners whose core ideas differ with each other. We suspect the rationale for this is often practical and compatible with guild rather than scientific interests.[16]

Psychodynamic psychiatry (the discipline), on the other hand, flatly rejects postmodernism. Its values are those of the enlightenment and fully compatible with those of science. (This is not to say that all of its beliefs and hypotheses have been scientifically validated, of course.)

Psychodynamic psychiatry therefore embraces only a part of the vast domain of psychoanalytic psychology. It includes that part of psychoanalysis that is directly clinically applicable and that part that borders on or is part of scientific knowledge.

Freud himself was concerned that his vast contributions would be reduced to the very segment of knowledge that psychodynamic psychiatry includes.[17]

In our view, accommodation with reality can be painful but is necessary for organized psychiatry to retain its vitally important psychodynamic component.

THE MODERN MEANING OF THE TERM *PSYCHOANALYSIS*

There is no central authority that defines the term *psychoanalysis* in a way that is universally acceptable. In our view, the term refers to selected ideas, many but not all of which were originally discovered by Freud. These can and should be specified as is convenient and necessary in clinical and scientific discussions of psychodynamics.

We suggest that contemporary articles in the area of psychodynamic psychiatry simply specify which core psychoanalytic ideas are referenced. This we suspect will diminish much confusion and increase specificity of discussions in the modern literature.

For example, an author might state (in a footnote): "In this article I discuss psychoanalytic ideas about male and female aspects of psychology. I refer to Freud's Three Essays on the Theory of Sexuality as well as more modern texts by X, Y and Z."

PSYCHODYNAMIC PSYCHIATRY AND MODERN KNOWLEDGE

Here we would especially include research and clinical publications pertaining to:

- Attachment theory
- Neuropsychiatry
- Sexual differentiation theory
- Neuropharmacology
- Endocrinology
- Genetics
- Trauma theory
- Coping and resilience

This is not an all-inclusive list but is of central importance in considering studies of treatment and of etiology of psychopathology.

SUMMARY

Psychodynamic psychiatry emerged from psychoanalytic theory, but the influence of the latter has been only partial. Equally important are other disciplines outlined above—especially biopsychological areas. Modern psychodynamic publications and presentations should honor all foundational pillars of the field. In this way, the new area lends itself to bio-psycho-social integrations that remain a challenge for all researchers and clinicians who seek to understand and treat patients with mental disorders.

REFERENCES

1. American Psychiatric Association. Diagnostic and statistical manual of mental disorders (DSM-II). 2nd edition. Washington, DC: American Psychiatric; 1968.
2. American Psychiatric Association. Diagnostic and statistical manual of mental disorders (DSM-III). 3rd edition. Washington, DC: American Psychiatric; 1968.
3. Hale NG. The rise and crisis of psychoanalysis in the United States. Bridgewater (NJ): Replica Books; 2000.
4. Engel GL. Psychological development in health and disease. Philadelphia: Saunders; 1964.
5. Breger L. Freud: darkness in the midst of vision. New York: Wiley; 2001.
6. Bayer RV. Homosexuality and American psychiatry: the politics of diagnosis. New York: Basic; 1981.
7. Friedman RC. Male homosexuality: a contemporary psychoanalytic perspective. New Haven (CT): Yale University Press; 1988.
8. Friedman RC, Downey JI. Biology and the oedipus complex. Psychoanal Q 1995; 64(2):234–64.
9. Phoenix CH, Goy RW, Gerall AA, et al. Organizing action of prenatally administered testosterone propionate on the tissues mediating mating behavior in the femal guinea pig. Endocrinology 1959;65:369–82.
10. Lacan J. The seminar of Jacques Lacan. The four fundamental concepts of psychoanalysis. New York: W. W. Norton & Company; 1973.
11. Jung CG. Psychological types. Princeton (NJ): Princeton University Press; 1971.
12. Jung CG, Hull RFC. The archetypes and the collective unconscious. London: Routledge & Paul; 1959.
13. Horney K. The neurotic personality of our time. New York: Norton & Company; 1994.

14. Auchincloss EL. The psychoanalytic model of the mind. Arlington (VA): American Psychiatric Publishing; 2015.
15. Freud S, Strachey J, Freud A, et al. The standard edition of the complete psychological works of Sigmund Freud. London: Hogarth Press; 1953.
16. Sokal A, Bricmont J. Fashionable nonsense: postmodern intellectuals' abuse of science. New York: Picador; 1998.
17. Freud S, Freud S. The problem of lay-analyses. New York: Brentano; 1927.

Preserving the Person in Contemporary Psychiatry

Glen O. Gabbard, MD

KEYWORDS

• Psychodynamic • Unconscious • Person • Transference • Countertransference • Resistance

KEY POINTS

- Psychodynamic psychiatry is defined by a way of thinking that involves a set of principles: unconscious mental functioning, transference, countertransference, resistance, the unique value of subjective experience, and the link between the past and the present.
- Contemporary psychiatry is at risk of losing the notion of "person" by emphasizing formal diagnosis.
- "Person" involves what is unique and idiosyncratic about an individual, whereas current psychiatric diagnosis involves common characteristics of a group of people that allow them to be placed in the same category.

Psychodynamic thinking has always been subversive. At its heart is the notion that we are consciously confused and unconsciously controlled. Its emphasis on subjectivity places it at odds with so-called hard science, which involves phenomena that are objective and measurable. Despite the long tradition of psychodynamic psychotherapy in mental health practice, there has been a hard fight for its survival. In both scientific publications and the news media, psychodynamic therapy is frequently contrasted with empirically validated treatments. Cognitive-behavioral therapy is often held up as the gold standard of the empirically validated therapies, whereas psychodynamic therapy is repeatedly identified as a form of treatment whose efficacy has not been established.

This state of affairs is finally changing. Steinert and colleagues[1] published a meta-analysis that tested equivalence of outcomes in psychotherapy using 23 randomized controlled trials with 2751 subjects included. The meta-analysis controlled for researcher allegiance effects by including both representatives of cognitive-behavioral therapy and psychodynamic therapy as investigators. The

Disclosure Statement: The author has no relationship with a commercial company that has a direct financial interest in the subject matter or materials discussed in this article or with a company making a competing product.

4306 Yoakum Boulevard, #535, Houston, TX 77006, USA
E-mail addresses: Glen.Gabbard@gmail.com; gg@glengabbard.com

Psychiatr Clin N Am 41 (2018) 183–191
https://doi.org/10.1016/j.psc.2018.01.001
psych.theclinics.com
0193-953X/18/

results, published in the *American Journal of Psychiatry*, suggested the equivalence of psychodynamic therapy to treatments established in efficacy.

To a large extent, the fate of psychodynamic psychiatry has been linked to the respect with which the modality has been regarded. However, although psychodynamic psychotherapy involves a specific set of technical interventions based on relevant theories, psychodynamic psychiatry is much broader. It involves a way of thinking about both patient and clinician.[2] This perspective can be applied to patients who would not be suitable for psychoanalysis or psychodynamic psychotherapy. Indeed, almost all patients seen by psychiatrists, no matter what the treatment, can be understood in psychodynamic terms, often integrated with information from the neurosciences. The type of thinking used in the context of psychodynamic psychiatry encompasses major psychoanalytic theories, such as object relations theory, self psychology, ego psychology, and relational or intersubjective theory; however, it also involves an understanding of the mind-brain connection. Psychodynamic psychiatry is essentially a biopsychosocial model that takes seriously influences from the environment and genes in understanding who the patient is. Nevertheless, certain guiding principles are at the core of this way of thinking:

- Unconscious mental functioning
- The unique value of the patient's subjective experience
- Past is prologue
- Transference
- Countertransference
- Resistance.

This set of principles can serve as a guide to clinicians as they listen to the patient's narrative and try to understand how the patient came to develop a unique identity like no other. The psychodynamic psychiatrist pursues the course often attributed to Hippocrates; that is, it is more important to know what sort of person has a disease than to know what sort of disease the person has.

Contemporary psychiatry is at risk of losing the notion of "person" in an era in which genomic data, brain scanning, and laboratory studies are valorized, whereas spending time with the patient is often regarded as time-inefficient. Fifteen-minute interviews for initial diagnostic assessment are widely used throughout North America, barring a truly in-depth evaluation. Moreover, the rise of the electronic medical record has created a situation in which eye contact between psychiatrist and patient may be minimized. In some cases, the clinician's absorption in the task of typing limits visual information about the patient to the beginning and the end of the interview.

The current emphasis in psychiatry places great importance on a formal diagnosis based on characteristics that are supposedly held in common by other patients with the same diagnosis. Hence, neuroimaging studies search for elements in the brain that would suggest a diagnostic category drawn from the official nomenclature of psychiatry. Preserving the "person" in psychiatry relies on a distinctly different approach. The core of that strategy is to let the patient tell his or her story so that what is unique and idiosyncratic about the individual emerges in a clinical assessment. As the diagnosis and treatment are pursued, the clinician is increasingly interested in determining how the patient may differ from others, more than how the patient is similar to those occupying a common diagnostic category.

One of the great ironies today is that the phrase personalized medicine connotes characteristics of the patient's genome rather than an understanding of the person. In fact, personalized medicine is a now popularized way of discussing the genetic characteristics of a patient. The true "person" with the illness is not a central focus. This narrow approach has created a backlash in both medicine and psychiatry circles. Horwitz and colleagues[3] have argued that even in nonpsychiatric illnesses, such as heart disease or diabetes, factors as stress, behavior, diet, and culture are likely to be more relevant than the patient's genome in determining risk. They have argued for a shift of emphasis that takes into account the environment of the patient, as well as the patient's personal attributes. Environmental factors have significant influence on the genomic expression. Experience leads to the laying down of neural networks that become the basis of self-image and expectations of how others will behave. Representations of people, objects, and situations are stored in the brain in the matrix of connections, that is, the synapses. These internalized phenomena serve as figures that haunt the individual throughout life. Finally, a major point relevant to this discussion is that monozygotic twins with identical genomes may be highly distinct individuals. In other words, personal identity does not necessarily overlap with genomic identity.[4]

Psychiatrists must be trained to recognize that they are diagnosing persons, not simply illnesses. Official diagnostic nomenclature in psychiatry plays a role but it is insufficient by itself to provide a thorough understanding that informs treatment following from the diagnosis.

THE SEARCH FOR THE PERSON

There was a time in psychiatric training in which the person was at the heart of the curriculum. *The Person*, by Theodore Lidz,[5] was widely read by medical students and psychiatric residents in the late 1960s and early 1970s. It traced the normal development of the person from birth through old age. Even in that era, the author warned that young physicians might become indifferent to patients as they became assimilated into the system of medical education. Retaining a notion of the person being examined was considered to be at the heart of good practice.

Today a psychiatric resident might be hard pressed to define exactly what is meant by "person" because the term has faded from contemporary discourse. Although it might be reasonable to simply use the term as a synonym for the self, such equivalence would not be entirely accurate. Philosophers such as Strawson[6] have pointed out that the word self is embedded in a context that involves religious, philosophic, psychological, and psychiatric perspectives that are heavily driven by theory and extremely diverse. If one considers psychoanalytic thinking, from which psychodynamic psychiatry derives, one is struck at the confusing usage throughout the literature on the self. It is often invoked to refer to an intrapsychic representation but is also commonly used to include a structure that subsumes experience or personal agency.[7–9] A further problem with equating "self" and "person" is that the self is both subject and object. Consider the following sentence: "I think of myself." In this sentence the self as the phenomenal "I" of philosophy is a part of the person who thinks about the self. On the other hand, in the word "myself" there is an implication that the self is a representation of something that can be objectified and thought about. So the 2 concepts of the self combined in this sentence illustrate both the subject and object roles of the self.

To complicate matters further, we certainly cannot limit the notion of the self to conscious contents of the mind. Psychodynamic therapy and psychoanalysis regularly reveal that shameful aspects of the self are repressed and split off to help us avoid unacceptable feelings that might be part of the human condition. In that regard, most of us are masters of self-deception who defend against certain aspects of ourselves.

Memory, of course, plays a significant role in the development of the self because narrative continuity depends on the aggregate of personal memories and the social personas that are associated with them.

The forgoing considerations lead us to the conclusion that the self is both a conscious and unconscious construct. Many choices we make, impulses we express, and thoughts that zip through our minds are reflecting disavowed parts of the self that are largely unconscious. Feelings often emerge that we cannot explain because they have been banned from our conscious view of the self and relegated to the nether-regions of the unconscious. The philosopher Thomas Nagel[10] made the point that we can use the term "I" to describe one's self even though our actual self-knowledge of who we are is confused and limited. To integrate the self into an understanding of the person may have some usefulness but we must certainly recognize the limitations. As psychotherapy often reveals, there is a mismatch between the way that we think, feel, and act, and the narrative we have internalized from childhood that bears the weight of our moral value system and our conscience. We regularly think quietly to ourselves, "I'm not acting like myself" or "This isn't like me."

This discussion of the self illustrates that the self-concept is far from monolithic. In fact, throughout psychoanalytic writing in the last several decades, it has become an accepted notion that we are all composed of multiple discontinuous selves that are constantly redefined and shaped by real and fantasized relationships with others. The notion of a continuous self is an illusion. Schafer[11] understood this phenomenon as a set of narrative selves or storylines that we develop to provide a coherent account of our lives. Mitchell[12] noted that a paradox of psychoanalytic work is that, as patients learn to tolerate multiple facets of themselves, they begin to experience themselves as more durable and more coherent. What we know as the self is context-dependent. Different aspects of the self are evoked by different individual and different group settings that are present in our environment.

Perhaps among the most influential contexts is the culture in which one grows up. A contemporary perspective on psychodynamic psychiatry must include ethnicity and culture as a primary factor in self-development. Gish Jen,[13] a Chinese novelist, emphasizes that Asian culture is not centered in self-experience. Rather, she asserts, an interdependent self is created by parenting that focuses on social context. Hence, a person steeped in an Asian upbringing is less likely to focus on the self-construct apart from its cultural and familial milieu.

SELF VERSUS PERSON

After this detour into the problem of the self in contemporary psychoanalytic thinking, returning to the person makes it clear that the self is not the same thing as the person. The writing about the self is generally linked to subjective experience; that is, reflecting on one's inner nature. However, one must contrast the self-as-experienced with the self-as-observed by others. The way that one is perceived by others allows for a fuller definition of the person. A useful example is how one reacts when seeing one's self on videotape. Most people who view themselves on video do not react positively to how they appear and sound on screen. In fact, most people are somewhat shocked when they see themselves on video because it contrasts, to a considerable degree, with how they imagine they appear and sound. When psychiatric residents view themselves interviewing a patient, common reactions include, "I don't look like that!" or "My voice doesn't sound like that!" Those in the same seminar with the resident will disagree and point out to the concerned colleague, "Yes, you actually do look like that and sound like that." The resident may be even more firm by asserting that, "I hear my voice all the time and it doesn't sound that way."

The humor in these situations in which one is startled about how they appear and sound leads to a significant issue in shaping who the person actually is. One could conduct a debate regarding whether the self as subjectively experienced is more valid than the self as observed by others. However, most would conclude that both constructs are important to a comprehensive view of the person. We simply do not see ourselves in the way that others see us no matter how hard we try.

Although an individual has difficulty ascertaining how others view him or her, it is also true that others who are observing from an outside perspective cannot see how the individual feels inside. A key point is that knowing who the person is requires integration of the inside and outside perspectives. In dynamic psychotherapy, a critically important aspect of the working through the process involves the therapy's shift from a first-person perspective, provided by the patient, to a third-person perspective emanating from the therapist.[14] In other words, therapists must empathically validate the patient's "I" experience, while also bringing to bear their own outside experience as an observer of the person.

Obstacles to Integrating Psychodynamic Psychiatry into Current Psychiatric Thinking

One of the major obstacles that long interfered with the inclusion of the person as part of the diagnostic understanding in psychiatry grew out of the official diagnostic nomenclature of the American Psychiatric Association. The *Diagnostic and Statistical Manual of Mental Disorders* (DSM)-III and DSM-IV classification system separated out an axis of personality disorders from another axis of diagnostic syndromes, such as anxiety, depression, schizophrenia, and so forth. Although the intent was to assure that a clinician diagnosing a patient would consider the personality dimensions of the patient, a clinician was prone to ignore the personality disorder axis all together. A frequent observation in that era on reviewing patient charts was that in the category under axis II, the word "deferred" often appeared. The assumption apparently was that at a later point the personality of the patient might be considered more thoroughly. However, in practice, the word "deferred" could easily have been replaced by "ignored."

A common experience of the attending working with psychiatric residents in that era was to hear a trainee use the following phrase: "I think this patient has some axis II stuff." Even though the DSM-5 system did away with the multiple axis system, one continues to hear the same phrase from young psychiatrists and trainees. The "axis II stuff" phrase was often code for "The patient is obnoxious, difficult, angry, manipulative, or otherwise unpleasant." Hence, the longstanding separation of personality disorder from syndrome in psychiatry led to a shorthand view that the patient with a diagnosis on axis II was antisocial, difficult, demanding, or unpleasant. The tendency to make this separation between personality and syndrome continues today despite the change in DSM-5. These broad brushstrokes tend to ignore dimensions of personality such as fear of disapproval, perfectionism, and dependency that are common elements of professionals such as psychiatrists. In the era of the "axis II stuff" the axis II label clearly was a pejorative adjective. Most germane to this article, however, is that it made it seem that the "person" was not relevant to the axis I diagnosis applied. In fact, it was common for trainees and young psychiatrists not to recognize the distinction between a personality disorder, on the 1 hand and the person, on the other.

Who Is the "Person?"

The foregoing overview of the problems inherent in integrating the notion of the person into contemporary psychiatry suggests that it is difficult to provide a simple categorization for that construct. Psychiatry is moving in the direction of rapid diagnosis based on symptom checklists; considering what is unique and idiosyncratic about the patient is viewed as too time-consuming. Incorporating the notion of the person into the teaching and practicing of psychiatry to make it truly psychodynamic-based involves a painstaking process of considering several different determinates that go into an understanding of who the patient is[2]:

1. The subjective experience of one's self based on a unique historical narrative that is filtered through the lens of specific meanings to the patient
2. A set of conscious and unconscious conflicts, defenses, representations, and self-deceptions
3. A set of internalized interactions with others that are unconsciously reenacted
4. One's physical characteristics
5. One's brain as a product of genes and interaction with environmental forces, and the creation of neural networks by cumulative experience
6. One's cultural or religious and social affiliations
7. One's cognitive style and cognitive capacities.

The inclusion of cognitive capacities and the integration of genetic factors with environmental forces are essential in this list of the determinants of personhood. In the contemporary mental health scene, psychodynamic thought must be integrated with biological forces to accurately diagnose the patient. A psychiatric diagnosis that ignores biology can be just as reductionist as one that ignores psychodynamic issues. There is no psychology without biology.

Case Example

The integration of the various factors that are involved in determining the person is complex and, at times, overwhelming. Clinicians must always approach the task with the expectation that the diagnostic understanding will be partial in the evaluation phase. As new material emerges in the course of treatment, one continues to alter the understanding based on that information. A case example may illustrate integrating diverse factors in a diagnostic assessment.

Ms A was a 44-year-old teacher who presented to treatment because of a recurrent depression that responded only partially to medication, feelings of self-depreciation, and a wish to improve her sexual desire in her marriage. She said that her husband was a good man and, therefore, she pretended to enjoy sex to please him. In fact, she had never had sexual desire throughout her life.

In her first session, I asked her to sit wherever she liked and she chose the chair that was farthest from my own chair. She asked me if I knew about the culture of the Hopi Indians. I told her I did not have much information about that culture but would like to hear what she had to say. Although she was not a product of the Hopi culture, she had studied it and informed me of a popular Hopi saying: "Each person finds the most appropriate seat for him or her when entering a room." I sensed she also needed some distance from me. That impression was confirmed when she told me a horrific childhood story about her incestuous relationship with her father from the age of 6 to 12 years. She found the abuse unbearably traumatic and said that she often found herself depersonalizing, floating above the bed, and dissociated from herself in such a way that she could view the abuse as occurring "to that girl down there" rather than to her. She kept the experience secret as she felt she could not discuss what was happening with her mother or with a friend. At 1 point she tried to tell a nun who taught her class in the Catholic school that she attended. The nun told her, "You must never speak of this again. You will burn in hell if you do." As a result, she developed a conviction that she was thoroughly bad.

As I got to know her, I recognized that her absence of sexual response or desire contributed to an ascetic self-view as one who does not need pleasure. She developed an identity as a self-disciplined long-distance runner who could take self-punishment with a stoic attitude. In this regard, one could integrate the psychological and biological elements of her condition using research on the impact of childhood sexual abuse. Heim and colleagues[15] studied a group of adult women who had been sexually abused as children and compared them with a control group who had not been abused. They found that exposure to childhood sexual abuse is specifically associated with cortical thinning in the area of the genital representation field within the primary somatosensory cortex. MRI scanning clearly showed this thinning in the portion of the brain associated with sexual feelings. In other words, the neuroplasticity associated with development seemed to protect the child from the sensory processing of specific abuse experiences but contributed to a deadening of the sexual response in adult life. Although on some level she understood that this was a situation that was unlikely to change, the patient felt that to be a good wife she should try to be more responsive to her husband. This absence of sexual response could be viewed as a deficit condition as opposed to a conflict-based problem in light of the neurologic modification associated with childhood sexual abuse. If it were to be viewed as a psychological conflict, then the patient might be expected to change this aspect of herself and feel like a failure for not being able to do so. Moreover, it might have contributed to her conviction that she was bad or defective in some way. This view was reinforced by religious-cultural factors in childhood, at least from her perspective, when the nun told her she must be secretive about what had happened to her. She later developed an altruistic devotion to teaching children and providing loving care for her 2 boys.

Ms A lived with the expectation that lightning would strike at any moment. Like many victims of childhood trauma, she harbored an assumption that positive expectations of others are dangerous because they might at any moment be shattered by aggression from others. Indeed she tended to redirect her rage at her parents toward herself through intense self-denigration. She also needed interpersonal distance, as shown at her choice of seating in my office. Finally, she had a tenacious clinging to suicidality as an escape hatch from the intolerable situation, even though she did not act on the suicidal thoughts.

In summary, the patient's sense of herself as a person, in my own observations as a psychodynamic psychiatrist trying to evaluate her, was that she had a confluence of early environmental factors and biological factors that led her to feel defective. She needed to come to terms with what was truly her fault versus those issues over which she had no control. The treatment plan had to take into account the limits of what one could expect given the alterations of cortical structures from the abuse.

Treatment Implications of Diagnosing the "Person"

One implication of this approach to diagnosis and treatment that integrates psychodynamic and psychiatric thinking is that we do not treat disorders in isolation. We are always treating a person with a disorder and this notion needs to be center stage in our planning. It is also true that the person and the therapist must be taken into account. Treatment is not simply a series of procedures that are geared to a specific diagnosis. We know that the therapeutic relationship seems to be far more important than a specific technique in predicting outcome.[16] The person of the therapist may be a good fit or a poor fit with the person of the patient. There is no doubt that the therapeutic alliance or therapeutic relationship may be enhanced if the fit is good and made more challenging if the fit is less than optimal.

One corollary to this notion of the importance of the therapeutic relationship is the capacity for the treating clinician to be flexible and shift his or her approach based on the patient's response. There is preliminary research suggesting that flexible shifting in the therapist's approach in response to the patient's characteristics is associated with better outcome.[17] The notion of optimal responsiveness seems to have an impact on outcome, meaning that the therapist who adjusts to what the patient needs may form a better therapeutic relationship that helps the patient improve as a result of the therapy process. Therapists who are flexible with the use of technique within a given treatment have better outcomes across their caseload compared with therapists who are much less flexible with their interventions. Therapists with the best outcomes, therefore, must adjust their approach based on their understanding of the particular patient's needs in the context of the treatment. The optimally responsive therapist is constantly monitoring his or her impact on the patient and modifying the approach so that it is as helpful as possible to a particular patient's needs, as well as acceptable to the patient's idiosyncratic ways of receiving help. In brief, therapeutic action must always take into account the unique features of the dyad.

There are a variety of reasons that the person is being ignored and neglected in contemporary psychiatry. There is a longing for simplicity, accompanied by a hatred of complexity, in many practitioners. Moreover, recognizing the patient in all of his or her complexity requires greater time and greater flexibility from the clinician. One might say that it is inconvenient. The simple fact is that getting to know the person takes time. As we all know in the current climate of practice, time is money. Technology has also contributed to the current resistance to seeing the uniqueness of the patient. As noted earlier, the requirement of typing while interviewing may actually decrease the time of face-to-face contact with the patient and, therefore, compromise empathy. Finally, getting to know the person in depth may be unsettling to the clinician. Facing a disturbed patient with a complex clinical picture may overwhelm an overworked clinician who may see 2 to 4 patients in an hour.

SUMMARY

Preserving the person in the diagnostic and treatment process of contemporary psychiatry involves a way of thinking that is time-consuming. Nevertheless, it may be far more gratifying than checking boxes on a short symptom checklist. Clinicians must let the patient tell his or her story in the time that is required. In this regard, we must also let the patient supervise us and lead us in the directions of his or her own uniqueness, even if the direction is counter to what we are developing in our own private formulation. We must constantly be thinking of integrating the biological, the psychological, and the sociocultural aspects of the patient. This task requires multiple visits over time and cannot be quickly accomplished. Nonetheless, even in the relatively brief appointments typical of today's psychiatric practice patterns, a point of view that emphasizes the person with the illness enriches the clinical encounter and understanding for both clinician and patient.

REFERENCES

1. Steinert C, Munder T, Rabung S, et al. Psychodynamic therapy: as efficacious as other empirically supported treatments? A meta-analysis testing equivalence of outcomes. Am J Psychiatry 2017;174(10):943–53.
2. Gabbard GO. Psychodynamic psychiatry in clinical practice. 5th edition. Arlington (VA): American Psychiatric Publishing Inc; 2014.

3. Horwitz RI, Cullen MR, Abell J, et al. (De) personalized medicine. Science 2013; 339:1155–6.
4. Mauron A. Personal identity. Science 2001;291:831–2.
5. Lidz T. The person: his development throughout the life cycle. New York: Basic Books; 1968.
6. Strawson G. Selves: revisionary metaphysics. Oxford (United Kingdom): Clarendon Press; 2009.
7. Kernberg OF. Self, ego, affects and drives. J Am Psychoanal Assoc 1982;30: 893–917.
8. Guntrip H. Schizoid phenomena, object-relations, and the self. New York: International Universities Press; 1968.
9. Sutherland JD. The British object relations theorists: Balint, Winnicott, Fairbairn, Guntrip. J Am Psychoanal Assoc 1980;28:829–60.
10. Nagel T. The view from nowhere. New York: Oxford University Press; 1986.
11. Schafer R. Retelling a life: narration and dialogue in psychoanalysis. New York: Basic Books; 1992.
12. Mitchell SA. Contemporary perspectives on self: toward an integration. Psa Dial 1991;1:121–47.
13. Jen G. Tiger writing: art, culture, and the interdependent self. Cambridge (MA): Harvard University Press; 2013.
14. Goldberg A. Between empathy and judgment. J Am Psychoanal Assoc 1999;47: 351–65.
15. Heim ZM, Mayberg HS, Mletzko T, et al. Decreased cortical representation of genital somatosensory field after childhood sexual abuse. Am J Psychiatry 2013;170:616–23.
16. Horvath AO. The therapeutic relationship: research and theory. An introduction to the special issue. Psychother Res 2005;15:3–7.
17. Owen J, Hilsenroth M. Treatment adherence: the importance of therapists' flexibility in relation to therapy outcomes. J Couns Psychol 2014;61:280–8.

The Place for Psychodynamic Therapy and Obstacles to Its Provision

Susan G. Lazar, MD[a,b,c,*]

KEYWORDS

- Psychodynamic treatment • Personality disorders • Chronic depressive disorders
- Anxiety disorders • Chronic complex disorders • Insurance company protocols
- Mental health parity

KEY POINTS

- Psychodynamic treatment has been shown to provide specific benefits for patients with personality disorders, chronic depressive and anxiety disorders, and chronic complex disorders, and its intensity and duration have independent positive effects.
- Obstacles to its provision include a bias privileging brief treatments, especially cognitive behavior therapy, seen as a gold standard of treatment, despite difficulties with the design and validity of, and the ability to generalize from, its supporting research and the diagnostic nosology of the illnesses studied.
- Another obstacle to the provision of psychodynamic psychotherapy lies in insurance company protocols that violate the mandate for mental health parity and focus on conserving insurers' costs rather than the provision of optimum treatment to patients.

Psychodynamic treatment has been shown to provide specific benefits for patients with personality disorders, chronic depressive and anxiety disorders, and chronic complex disorders, and its intensity and duration have independent positive effects. Obstacles to its provision include a bias privileging brief treatments, especially cognitive behavior therapy (CBT), seen as a gold standard of treatment, despite difficulties with the design and validity of, and the ability to generalize from, its supporting research and the diagnostic nosology of the illnesses studied. Another obstacle to the provision of psychodynamic psychotherapy lies in insurance company protocols that violate the mandate for mental health parity and focus on conserving insurers' costs rather than the provision of optimum treatment to patients.

[a] George Washington University School of Medicine, Washington, DC 20037, USA; [b] Uniformed Services University of the Health Sciences, Bethesda, MD, USA; [c] Washington Psychoanalytic Institute, Washington, DC 20037, USA
* 9104 Quintana Drive, Bethesda, MD 20817.
E-mail address: sglmd@aol.com

Psychiatr Clin N Am 41 (2018) 193–205
https://doi.org/10.1016/j.psc.2018.01.004

Those valuing short-term cost saving objectives more than optimum treatment might prefer to provide lower cost medication treatment. Nonetheless, psychotherapy is preferred to medication by 75% of patients,[1] often provides a greater effect size than medication alone, augments the effect of medication (although the reverse of medication augmenting psychotherapy is not established), has lower dropout rates than medication-alone protocols, and obviously lacks the side effects of medication treatments.[2]

Although psychotherapy for different approaches is effective for many patients, there is a common assumption that CBT is the superior and preferred approach. However, a recent study[3] showed psychodynamic therapy to be equivalent to other treatments established as efficacious. In addition, Leichsenring and Steinert,[4] 2017, challenge the gold-standard status of CBT with their findings of publication bias, its frequent small effect size, the influence of researcher allegiance, several meta-analyses revealing its limited efficacy, and response and remission rates of 50% or less for depression and anxiety leaving a large percentage of patients with insufficient improvement.

LENGTH AND INTENSITY OF PSYCHOTHERAPY

With respect to treatment "dosage," recent studies identify several diagnostic groups of patients who need an intensive and longer duration of psychotherapy, including those with chronic, debilitating personality disorders; chronic, complex disorders such as severe long-standing depression and anxiety; and multiple chronic psychiatric disorders. Among the most seriously ill, these patients are frequently not adequately treated with psychotherapy because of arbitrary limits on reimbursement for psychotherapy by insurance companies.[5] Patients with personality disorders are very costly to society; are among the most chronically impaired groups in psychiatric populations; are unemployed for long periods; and have high rates of drug problems, suicide attempts, interpersonal difficulties,[6–9] criminal behavior, divorce, child abuse, and heavy use of mental and general health care.[10] The lifetime prevalence of personality disorders is between 10% and 13.5%,[9,11–14] affecting 30 million Americans of all social classes, races, and ethnicities.

For these patients who need more psychotherapy, both longer duration and higher frequency of psychotherapy have independent positive effects and contribute to the most positive treatment outcomes.[15–19] The cost-effectiveness and cost offset of extended intensive psychotherapy for those patients who need it include savings from decreased sick leave, and decreased medical costs and decreased hospital costs.[20–30]

Patients with borderline personality disorder (BPD) take significantly longer to improve.[31–36] The British Health Service National Institute for Health and Care Excellence cautions against brief psychological interventions for BPD, stating, "...there is perhaps an even stronger signal that longer treatments with higher doses are of greater benefit. In several studies, significant improvement was only observed after 12 months of active treatment."[37(p207)]

Depression has a lifetime prevalence in the United States of 19.3% with major depression being a common diagnosis affecting 16.6% of adults,[38] occurring in 1 of every 10 to 20 primary care patients,[39] and is the most common diagnosis made in primary care.[40] Depression is experienced by one-fifth of all Americans at some point during their lifetimes,[41] and is extremely costly to society in increased medical costs, suicide-related mortality costs, and disability. A World Health Organization study[42] found unipolar depressive disorders to be the greatest cause of worldwide disability.

The 20% of depressed patients who are treatment resistant fare better with longer psychotherapy. Compared with other depressed patients, the treatment resistant have greater health care costs; are twice as likely to be hospitalized both for depression and general medical admissions; and have 12% more outpatient visits, 1.4 to 3 times more psychotropic medications, more than 6 times the mean total medical costs, and 19 times greater total depression-related costs.[43]

SPECIFIC EFFECTS OF PSYCHODYNAMIC PSYCHOTHERAPY

Psychodynamic therapy provides a specific advantage for patients with personality disorders and other chronic complex disorders who often have ingrained, inflexible, maladaptive ways of thinking and behaving leading to impaired relationships that constitute a highly significant risk factor for increased mortality exceeding smoking, alcoholism, obesity, and hypertension.[44] Although psychotherapy for different approaches improves symptoms, studies show that long-term psychodynamic treatments are significantly superior in improving maladaptive interpersonal relationships.[2,18,19,45–47] Compared with patients treated with other psychotherapies, patients treated with psychodynamic psychotherapy maintain therapeutic gains better and continue to improve after treatment ends; the so-called sleeper effect.[47]

For patients with BPD, one study[48] found no evidence that the core disorders of patients with BPD (unstable relationships, primitive defenses, identity disorder, and boredom) are affected by 1 year of dialectical behavior therapy (DBT). Several studies have found that dynamic psychotherapy leads to broader personality changes than supportive psychotherapy or DBT for BPD.[29,46]

Perfectionistic depressed patients also need more than a brief course of psychotherapy and do better with intensive extended psychodynamic therapy.[49,50] For depressed patients with residual symptoms after treatment, a literature review of unsatisfactory degrees of remission found that subsyndromal residual depressive symptoms can progress to prodromal symptoms of recurrence and may be the most consistent predictors of relapse.[51] Judging a patient successfully treated because of no longer meeting syndromal criteria of illness does not connote full recovery; residual symptoms may indicate the need for more extended treatment. Dysfunctional social and interpersonal patterns are also correlated with persistent depression, relapse, and poor long-term prognosis. Psychodynamic treatment is more effective for these traits that put patients at risk for recurring illness.[18,29,45–47]

Both a psychodynamic approach and the greater intensity of a psychoanalytic schedule add benefit for patients with unipolar depression. Long-term CBT, psychoanalytic therapies, and psychodynamic therapies yield similar improvements in depressive symptoms for all 3 approaches immediately after treatment. CBT and psychodynamic therapy patients have similar levels of depressive symptoms at 3-year follow-up. However, patients treated with the more intensive psychoanalytic treatment sustain greater improvement both in general distress and interpersonal problems immediately after treatment, and in depressive symptoms, general distress, interpersonal problems, and self-schema than the CBT group at 3-year follow-up.[45] Demonstrating the impact on the brain of the improvement in depression after long-term psychodynamic psychotherapy, Buchheim and colleagues[52] (2012) published the first study documenting its treatment-specific changes in the limbic system and regulatory regions in the prefrontal cortex.

Comorbidity is a frequent serious complication for depressive illness. Depressed patients with comorbid personality disorders have more treatment-resistant, persistent, and recurrent depression; role limitations; and impaired social functioning and health perceptions than patients with major depressive disorder alone. Depressed patients whose personality disorders remit improve in social functioning and have a likelier remittance of depression than those with persisting personality disorders, the group that functions the poorest. Depressed patients with comorbid personality disorders also have a longer time to achieve remission than depressed patients without personality disorders. Borderline and obsessive-compulsive personality disorders at baseline are robust predictors of accelerated relapse after remission from an episode of major depressive disorder, even controlling for other negative prognostic predictors. BPD is a robust independent predictor of chronicity (accounting for approximately 57% of persistent cases) and is the strongest predictor of persistence of major depressive disorder, followed by schizoid and schizotypal personality disorder, any anxiety disorder (the strongest axis I predictor), and dysthymic disorder.[53,54] Patients with major depression and a comorbid personality disorder need both illnesses treated to avoid recurrent and persistent depressive illness even when a longer and more intensive treatment is required.[55,56] As noted, psychodynamic treatments have a greater potential to ameliorate the perfectionism of many depressed patients, the disturbed interpersonal relations for those with personality disorders and other chronic conditions, and the core psychopathology of patients with BPD.

Other studies have examined outcome and cost-effectiveness for more than 5000 outpatients with a variety of common Diagnostic and Statistical Manual of Mental Disorders, Fourth Edition (DSM-4) axis 1 and 2 diagnoses treated with either long-term psychodynamic psychotherapy (LTPP) or psychoanalytic treatment. Both LTPP and psychoanalysis yield large effect sizes for symptom reduction, personality change, improvement in moderate disorders both at termination and follow-up, as well as reduced health care use and sick leave.[57,58] Psychoanalysis, with its greater frequency, is more costly but more cost-effective than LTPP from a health-related quality perspective[59,60] and both treatments yield significantly reduced work absenteeism and hospitalization at 7-year follow-up.[61]

Psychodynamic psychotherapies have also been found to be effective for anxiety disorders, eating disorders, substance abuse, somatic symptoms, and marital discord.[2]

THE OBSTACLES

Shortcomings in Nosology and Ability to Generalize Research

Evidence-supported psychotherapy is based on research studies of specific groups of patients generally with 1 Diagnostic and Statistical Manual of Mental Disorders (DSM) diagnosis. Since DSM-3 in 1980, psychiatric diagnosis has been based on observable symptoms not reflecting underlying chronic vulnerabilities that lead to recurrent symptoms and subjective distress. Much of this research focuses on brief, highly scripted forms of psychotherapy, studied in randomized controlled trials with subjects bearing a single DSM diagnosis without comorbidities. Brief therapies yielding statistically significant effects are promoted as the approaches of choice for the diagnoses studied. They do not identify efficacious therapies for most psychiatric patients because most have more complex conditions and comorbidity than those accepted into research cohorts, as, for example, the large population of patients with major depression (major depressive disorder), of whom 78.5% have additional psychiatric comorbidity with major depressive disorder not even their primary diagnosis.[41]

A finding of statistically significant reduction in symptoms does not necessarily signify meaningful, lasting improvement or recovery from illness. An extensive review of manualized brief treatments for depressive and anxiety disorders found that treatment benefits were short-lived; more than half of the patients in their sample sought treatment again within 6 to 12 months.[62] In addition, examinations of the research literature on randomized controlled trials for anxiety and depression[63] and on CBT for depression[64] found study design flaws and publication bias that undermined ostensible findings of efficacy. The findings of much academic research are often neither relevant to the clinical needs of patients nor appropriate information to shape health care policy or insurance company medical necessity protocols.

Underlying their acute symptoms, most psychiatric patients have chronic illnesses that often lead to repeated episodes of treatment. To be treated more definitively with psychotherapy, most need more than brief treatment with a primary focus on an acute presenting symptom. Many patients need ongoing psychotherapy or remain at risk of substance abuse, physical illness, and destructive behavior costly to themselves and to society. According to Shedler[65] (2015), brief, "'evidence-based' therapies are ineffective for most people most of the time."[65(p48)] Shedler[65] also quotes Driessen and colleagues[66] (2013) with regard to a study of depressed patients treated with brief CBT or psychodynamic therapy: "Our findings indicate that a substantial proportion of patients....require more than time-limited therapy to achieve remission."66[(p1047)] In sum, 75% of patients did not get well.

If diagnostic schemes are descriptive of different superficial observable symptoms and overlooking more salient commonalities between them, what more accurate and nuanced concepts would identify and focus treatment on the underlying drivers of illness? In examining patterns of comorbidity among common mental disorders, Krueger[67] (1999) conceives of them not as discrete, dichotomous entities, but rather as "extreme points on continua that span a range of emotional and behavioral functioning."[67(p922)] Superficial nosology accounts in large measure for the frequent finding of "comorbidity."

Brown and colleagues[68] (1998) noted that "the expansion of our nosologies has come at the expense of less empirical consideration of shared or overlapping features of emotional disorders that...may have far greater significance in the understanding of the prevention, etiology, and course of disorders, and in predicting their response to treatment...Our classification systems have become overly precise to the point that they are now erroneously distinguishing symptoms and disorders that actually reflect inconsequential variations of broader, underlying syndromes."[68(p179)]

Several researchers have focused on delineating common variables shared by certain diagnostic categories. Watson and Clark[69] (1984) and Brown and colleagues[68] (1998) note negative affect as a construct connecting patients with symptoms of anxiety and depression. Barlow and colleagues[70] (2014) postulate neuroticism as a common factor among anxiety and related disorders and their high rate of comorbidity. Krueger and colleagues[71] (2001) link dimensions of mental disorder with dimensions of personality, with, for example, internalization (linked with higher negative emotionality) and externalization (linked with lower constraint.)

Two other promising approaches are intended to provide a more in-depth and accurate assessment and guide to treatment of mental disorders. The Psychodynamic Diagnostic Manual, which assesses the level of personality organization, quality of mental functioning, and subjective experience of symptoms,[72] is a comprehensive psychodynamic diagnostic tool that provides a detailed assessment of psychological strengths and vulnerabilities. The resultant profile yields a more nuanced and specific diagnosis of a patient's psychiatric illness than designations of superficial and observable symptoms. Another is the study of patients' level and quality of mentalization,[73] which are assessed along several axes to examine the maturity of the patient's capacity to make sense of the patient's own subjective states and mental processes as well as those of others. The maturity of a patient's mentalization is seen as a driving factor in psychiatric illness, as the appropriate focus of psychotherapy, and its improvement is seen as the signal indicator of a treatment's success.

INSURANCE COMPANY OBSTACLES TO PROVISION OF ADEQUATE PSYCHOTHERAPY

Insurance Protocols, Medical Necessity, and Utilization Review

Given decades of stigma and lack of appropriate support for psychotherapy and all mental health care, most psychiatric illness is still undiagnosed and untreated or inadequately treated.[74–76] The lack of sufficient treatment is a hidden multiplier of morbidity, disability, and greatly expanded overall health care expenses for patients with psychiatric illness compared with those without psychiatric illness. The increased medical expenses of the psychiatrically ill go beyond the costs of their psychiatric care and include more primary care visits, higher outpatient charges, and longer hospital stays.[75,77,78]

If inadequately treated, large patient groups are very costly to society and often need more intensive and/or extended psychotherapy than most insurance companies are willing to support, despite research documenting the cost-effectiveness of an appropriate level of care to achieve recovery and savings that often result from their decreased medical expenses and improved productivity. Insurance companies focus on controlling their short-term costs and not on thorough treatment that leads to better health outcomes and savings over time in the budgets of other parties. According to the US Department of Labor Bureau of Labor Statistics 2016 report,[79] the median number of years that wage and salary workers had been with their current employer declined to 4.2 years in January 2016, down from 4.6 years in January 2014. Thus, subscribers who obtain medical insurance through their employers change their insurance providers every few years. The cost savings by under-reimbursing mental health care are of greater interest to an insurer; a cost offset in overall medical expenses in the future by virtue of the adequate coverage of mental health services would not be a consideration to a current insurer focused on its own immediate expenses. An insurer's preferential support for very brief courses of psychotherapy undermines the provision of extended and intensive psychodynamic therapy for the patients who need it for optimum recovery.

Insurers also perpetuate stigma against psychotherapy in their concern that readily available outpatient psychotherapy would be overused. However, a RAND study showed that when weekly outpatient psychotherapy is fully covered, only 4.3% of the insured population uses it and the average length of treatment is 11 sessions.[80] With respect to those patients who need more, a long history of higher copayments for mental health services reduces both initial access to and treatment intensity of mental health visits, and this reduction of care affects patients at all levels of clinical need.[81,82] A more recent study found that increasing costs to patients for mental health care leads to a significant decrease in new mental health visits in equal measure for both severe and mild disorders but a larger decrease in low-income compared with high-income neighborhoods. Furthermore, the costs of an associated increase in involuntary commitment and acute mental health care exceed the cost savings from the decline in new mental health visits. Increasing costs to patients reduces access to mental health care and increases costs and morbidity, particularly among high-need, vulnerable populations.[83,84] Poor and very ill psychiatric patients are disproportionately affected by discriminatory copayments and financial disincentives designed to screen out a hypothetical group of patients who it is feared would capriciously abuse covered mental health services.[85]

MEDICAL NECESSITY AND UTILIZATION REVIEW

The concept of medical necessity is central to managed care and used routinely by insurers to evaluate medical claims eligible for reimbursement.[86] Although The Mental Health Parity and Addiction Equity Act (MHPAEA) of 2008 requires health insurers to use equivalent standards to authorize and provide the same levels of coverage for mental health care as for other medical conditions (parity), health insurers use much more limited definitions of medical necessity for mental health treatment than for other medical care. A 2003 report by the Substance Abuse and Mental Health Services Administration (SAMHSA[87]) found that medical necessity criteria are generally designed by insurers, not treating clinicians, and are used to limit reimbursement for treatments deemed inconsistent with insurers' interpretations of relative cost and efficiency, even when care is demonstrably consistent with professional standards. The SAMHSA report found that neither state nor federal regulatory processes universally controlled medical necessity standards promulgated by insurers.[88]

Although the Mental Health Parity Act did not alter insurers' control of criteria for medical necessity, it mandated public disclosure of their clinical standards,[89] an action consistent with the recommendations of the Institute of Medicine (IOM).[90] In 2011, after the passage of the Affordable Care Act (ACA) and its mandate of essential health benefits (which includes mental health care and psychotherapy among its components), the American Medical Association (AMA) issued a public statement to the IOM Committee on Determination of Essential Health Benefits[91] defining medical necessity as:

> *Health care services or products that a prudent physician would provide to a patient for the purpose of preventing, diagnosing or treating an illness, injury, disease or its symptoms in a manner that is (a) in accordance with generally accepted standards of medical practice; (b) clinically appropriate in terms of type, frequency, extent, site and duration; and (c) not primarily for the economic benefit of the health plans and purchases or for the convenience of the patients, treating physician, or other health care provider.*

The AMA statement reiterated the mandate for parity of coverage for all essential health benefits (which include mental health care.) This AMA definition was endorsed in a 2015 official position statement by the American Psychiatric Association (APA).[92]

Although most insurance plans ostensibly incorporate these AMA and APA position statements on medical necessity, many managed behavioral health care organizations create medical necessity criteria grossly at odds with them. This disturbing, frequently unchallenged practice often takes the form of proprietary medical necessity criteria claiming consistency with generally accepted standards of medical practice but categorically failing to address the chronicity and pervasiveness of mental illnesses and substance use disorders. They also apportion inadequate care based on a false premise that the generally accepted standard for psychiatric care is to focus solely on time-limited treatment of acute symptoms until their resolution to the condition before their onset. For example, several national managed behavioral health care organizations have used proprietary medical necessity criteria that expressly define outpatient treatment as acute and require acute symptoms to justify its provision. Their standards also ignore data in professional guidelines (cited as references for their own guidelines) about the need for extended and intensive psychotherapy for chronic conditions.

Contrary to both generally accepted standards of medical practice and mental health parity laws, proprietary guidelines commonly require objective proof that psychiatric illness will deteriorate in the absence of proposed care or that less expensive, potentially inferior treatments have not worked or will not work. To demand a less intensive treatment to fail first devalues the clinical judgment of treating providers and imposes unacceptable risks on mental health care that are not tolerated in the medical/surgical context. As noted in the American Society of Addiction Medicine criteria,[93] a "treatment failure" approach puts the patient at risk by delaying a more definitive level of treatment and potentially increasing health care costs by allowing the addictive disorder to progress. "Fail-first" policies are also demoralizing to patients who are made to feel untreatable when they are being inadequately treated.

Utilization review is an insurance company's monitoring process to pre-authorize reimbursement for recommended treatment and to assess with "clinical reviews" ongoing treatments for continuing eligibility for reimbursement. In violation of mental health parity, utilization review is used more restrictively for mental health treatment than for other medical care for both preauthorization of new care and clinical review of ongoing treatment. Clinical review protocols often stop coverage for a course of mental health treatment when acute symptoms have improved to a patient's baseline condition without resolving chronic underlying vulnerabilities to repeated episodes of acute illness.[94]

Utilization review has been found to lack reliability and validity, to impose a needless administrative burden, and to cause a sentinel effect in which providers experience a distortion in their practice style from the expectation of intrusive insurance company review. Very brief psychotherapy is often authorized for a broad spectrum of diagnoses regardless of severity.[95]

Medical necessity and utilization review protocols are too often designed to conserve insurance company costs in the short term without consideration of the sequelae from undertreated illness: its increased associated costs in other medical services, in increased morbidity and mortality, and the enormous costs to society in increased disability.[93–95]

Given appropriate medical necessity guidelines at parity with other medical care, consistent with provider expertise and a broad range of psychotherapy research, there would be no need or place for utilization review protocols. The national goal should be mental health parity without the interference of insurers' cost and profit concerns undermining the provision of appropriate care. Frequency and duration of psychotherapy as prescribed by the clinician should be supported without arbitrary limitations.

ACKNOWLEDGMENTS

The author would like to acknowledge the invaluable suggestions of Glen Gabbard, Jonathan Shedler, Nancy McWilliams, Kenneth Levy, Frank Yeomans, Eric Plakun, and Meiram Bendat.

REFERENCES

1. McHugh RK, Whitton SW, Peckham AD, et al. Patient preference for psychological vs pharmacologic treatment of psychiatric disorders: a meta-analytic review. J Clin Psychiatry 2013;74:595–602.
2. Levy KN, Ehrenthal JC, Yeomans FE, et al. Efficacy of psychotherapy: psychodynamic psychotherapy as an example. Psychodyn Psychiatry 2014;42:377–422.
3. Steinert C, Munder T, Rabung S, et al. Psychodynamic therapy: as efficacious as other empirically supported treatments? A meta-analysis testing equivalence of outcomes. Am J Psychiatry 2017;174(10):943–53.

4. Leichsenring F, Steinert C. Is cognitive behavioral therapy the gold standard for psychotherapy?: the need for plurality in treatment and research. JAMA 2017; 318(14):1323–4.
5. Bendat M. In name only? Mental health parity or illusory reform. Psychodyn Psychiatry 2014;42(3):353–75.
6. Gabbard GO. Psychotherapy of personality disorders. J Psychother Pract Res 2000;9(1):1–6.
7. Linehan MM, Heard HI. Borderline personality disorder. In: Miller NE, Magruder KM, editors. Cost effectiveness of psychotherapy. New York: Oxford University Press; 1999. p. 291–305.
8. Pilkonis PA, Neighbors BD, Corbitt EM. Personality disorders. In: Miller NE, Magruder KM, editors. Cost-effectiveness of psychotherapy. New York: Oxford University Press; 1999. p. 279290.
9. Reich J, Yates W, Nduaguba M. Prevalence of DSM-III personality disorders in the community. Soc Psychiatry Psychiatr Epidemiol 1989;24(1):12–6.
10. Skodol AE, Gunderson JG, Shea MT, et al. The collaborative longitudinal personality disorders study (CLPS): Overview and implications. J Personal Disord 2005; 19(5):487–504.
11. Casey PR, Tyrer PJ. Personality, functioning and symptomatology. J Psychiatr Res 1986;20(4):363–74.
12. Maier W, Lichtermann D, Klingler T, et al. Prevalences of personality disorders (DSM-III-R) in the community. J Personal Disord 1992;6(3):187–96.
13. Zimmerman M, Coryell WH. Diagnosing personality disorders in the community: a comparison of self-report and interview measures. Arch Gen Psychiatry 1990; 47(6):527–31.
14. Lenzenweger MF. Epidemiology of personality disorders. Psychiatr Clin North Am 2008;31(3):395–403.
15. Rudolf G, Manz R, Ori C. Ergebnisse psychoanalytischer therapie. [Outcome of psychoanalytic therapy]. Z Psychosom Med Psychother 1994;40:25–40.
16. Sandell R, Blomberg J, Lazar A, et al. Varieties of long-term outcome among patients in psychoanalysis and longterm psychotherapy: a review of findings in the Stockholm Outcome of Psychoanalysis and Psychotherapy Project (STOPPP). Int J Psychoanal 2000;81:921–42.
17. Grande T, Dilg R, Jakobsen T, et al. Differential effects of two forms of psychoanalytic therapy: results of the Heidelberg-Berlin study. Psychother Res 2006;16(4): 470–85.
18. Leichsenring F, Rabung S. Effectiveness of long-term psychodynamic psychotherapy: a meta-analysis. J Am Med Assoc 2008;300(13):1551–65.
19. Leichsenring F, Rabung S. Long-term psychodynamic psychotherapy in complex mental disorders: update of a meta-analysis. Br J Psychiatry 2011;199(1):15–22.
20. Düehrssen A. Katamnestische Ergebnisse bei 1004 Patienten nach analytischer Psychotherapie. Zeitschrift für psychosomatische Medizin 1962;8:94–113.
21. Heinzel R, Breyer F, Klein T. Ambulante Psychoanalyse in Deutschland: Eine katamnestische evaluation studie (No. 281), Diskussionsbeiträge: Serie 1. Baden-Wurtemmberg (Germany): Fakultät für Wirtschaftswissenschaften und Statistik, Universität Konstanz; 1996.
22. Dossmann R, Kutter P, Heinzel R, et al. The long-term benefits of intensive psychotherapy: a view from Germany. Psychoanalytic Inq 1997;17(S1):74–86
23. Keller W, Westhoff G, Dilg R, et al. Efficacy and cost effectiveness aspects of outpatient (Jungian) psychoanalysis and psychotherapy—A catamnestic study. In: Leuzinger-Bohleber M, Target M, editors. Outcomes of psychoanalytic

treatment: Perspectives for therapists and researchers. London: Whurr Publishers; 1998. p. 186–200.
24. Bateman AW, Fonagy P. Effectiveness of partial hospitalization in the treatment of borderline personality disorder: a randomized controlled trial. Am J Psychiatry 1999;156(10):1563–9.
25. Hall J, Caleo S, Stevenson J, et al. An economic analysis of psychotherapy for borderline personality disorder patients. J Ment Health Policy Econ 2001;4(1): 3–8.
26. Bateman AW, Fonagy P. Health service utilization costs for borderline personality disorder patients treated with psychoanalytically oriented partial hospitalization versus general psychiatric care. Am J Psychiatry 2003;160(1):169–71.
27. Bateman A, Fonagy P. 8-year follow-up of patients treated for borderline personality disorder: mentalization-based treatment versus treatment as usual. Am J Psychiatry 2008;165(5):631–8.
28. Clarkin JF, Foelsch PA, Levy KN, et al. The development of a psychodynamic treatment for patients with borderline personality disorder: a preliminary study of behavioral change. J Personal Disord 2001;15(6):487–95.
29. Clarkin J, Levy K, Lenzenweger M, et al. Evaluating three treatments for borderline personality disorder: a multiwave study. Am J Psychiatry 2007;164(6):922–8.
30. van Asselt AD, Dirksen CD, Arntz A, et al. Out-patient psychotherapy for borderline personality disorder: cost-effectiveness of schema-focused therapy v. transference-focused psychotherapy. Br J Psychiatry 2008;192(6):450–7.
31. Howard KI, Kopta SM, Krause MS, et al. The dose-effect relationship in psychotherapy. Am Psychol 1986;41(2):159–64.
32. Høglend P. Personality disorders and long-term outcome after brief dynamic psychotherapy. J Personal Disord 1993;7(2):168–81.
33. Kopta SM, Howard KI, Lowry JL, et al. Patterns of symptomatic recovery in psychotherapy. J Consult Clin Psychol 1994;62(5):1009–16.
34. Seligman ME. The effectiveness of psychotherapy. The Consumer Reports study. Am Psychol 1995;50(12):965–74.
35. Fonagy P, editor. An open door review of outcome studies in psychoanalysis. 2nd edition. London: International Psychoanalytical Association; 2002.
36. Levy KN, Meehan KB, Yeomans FE. Transference-focused psychotherapy reduces treatment drop-out and suicide attempters compared with community psychotherapist treatment in borderline personality disorder. Evid Based Ment Health 2010;13:119.
37. National Institute for Health and Care Excellence (NICE). Borderline personality disorder: treatment and management. P.207 NICE Clinical Guideline 78. London (UK): Department of Health; 2009.
38. Kessler RC, Berglund P, Demler O, et al. Lifetime prevalence and age-of-onset distributions of DSM-IV disorders in the National Comorbidity Survey Replication. Arch Gen Psychiatry 2005;62(6):593–602.
39. Halaris A. A primary care focus on the diagnosis and treatment of major depressive disorder in adults. J Psychiatr Pract 2011;17(5):340–50.
40. Katon W, Sullivan MD. Depression and chronic medical illness. J Clin Psychiatry 1990;51(Suppl):3–11.
41. Kessler RC, Berglund P, Demler O, et al. The epidemiology of major depressive disorder: results from the National Comorbidity Survey Replication (NCS-R). JAMA 2003;289(23):3095–105.
42. World Health Organization. The global burden of disease. Geneva (Switzerland): World Health Organization; 2008. ISBN: 978 92 4 156371 0.

43. Crown WH, Finkelstein S, Berndt ER, et al. The impact of treatment-resistant depression on health care utilization and costs. J Clin Psychiatry 2002;63:963–71.
44. Holt-Lunstad J, Smith TB, Layton JB. Social relationships and mortality risk: a meta-analytic review. PLoS Med 2010;7:e1000316.
45. Huber D, Zimmermann J, Henrich G, et al. Comparison of cognitive-behaviour therapy with psychoanalytic and psychodynamic therapy for depressed patients: a three-year follow-up study. Z Psychosom Med Psychother 2012;58(3):299–316.
46. Levy KN, Meehan KB, Kelly KM, et al. Change in attachment patterns and reflective function in a randomized control trial of transference-focused psychotherapy for borderline personality disorder. J Consult Clin Psychol 2006;74(6):1027–40.
47. Shedler J. The efficacy of psychodynamic psychotherapy. Am Psychol 2010;65: 98–109.
48. van den Bosch L, Verheul R, Schippers GM, et al. Dialectical behavior therapy of borderline patients with and without substance use problems: Implementation and long-term effects. Addict Behav 2002;27(6):911–23.
49. Blatt SJ. The differential effect of psychotherapy and psychoanalysis with anaclitic and introjective patients: the Menninger Psychotherapy-Research Project revisited. J Am Psychoanal Assoc 1992;40(3):691724.
50. Blatt SJ, Quinlan DM, Pilkonis PA, et al. Impact of perfectionism and need for approval on the brief treatment of depression: the National Institute of Mental Health Treatment of Depression Collaborative Research Program revisited. J Consult Clin Psychol 1995;63(1):125–32.
51. Fava GA, Ruini C, Belaise C. The concept of recovery in major depression. Psychol Med 2007;37(3):307–18.
52. Buchheim A, Viviani R, Kessler H, et al. Changes in prefrontal-limbic function in major depression after 15 months of long-term psychotherapy. PLoS One 2012; 7(3). https://doi.org/10.1371/journal.pone.0033745.
53. Grilo CM, Stout RL, Markowitz JC, et al. An episode of major depressive disorder: a 6-year prospective study. J Clin Psychiatry 2010;71(12):1629–35.
54. Skodol AE, Grilo CM, Keyes KM, et al. Relationship of personality disorders to the course of major depressive disorder in a nationally representative sample. Am J Psychiatry 2011;168(3):257–64.
55. Skodol AE, Grilo CM, Pagano ME, et al. Effects of personality disorders on functioning and well-being in major depressive disorder. J Psychiatr Pract 2005;11(6): 363–8.
56. Markowitz JC, Skodol AE, Petkova E, et al. Longitudinal effects of personality disorders on psychosocial functioning of patients with major depressive disorder. J Clin Psychiatry 2007;68(2):186–93.
57. De Maat S, Philipszoon F, Schoevers R, et al. Costs and benefits of long-term psychoanalytic therapy: changes in health care use and work impairment. Harv Rev Psychiatry 2007;15(6):289–300.
58. De Maat S, de Jonghe F, Schoevers R, et al. The effectiveness of long-term psychoanalytic therapy: a systematic review of empirical studies. Harv Rev Psychiatry 2009;17(1):1–23.
59. Berghout CC, Zevalkink J, Hakkaart-van Roijen L. A cost-utility analysis of psychoanalysis versus psychoanalytic psychotherapy. Int J Technol Assess Health Care 2010;26(1):3–10.
60. Berghout CC, Zevalkink J, Hakkaart-Van Roijen L. The effects of long-term psychoanalytic treatment on healthcare utilization and work impairment and their associated costs. J Psychiatr Pract 2010;16(4):209–16.

61. Beutel ME, Rasting M, Stuhr U, et al. Assessing the impact of psychoanalyses and long-term psychoanalytic therapies on health care utilization and costs. Psychother Res 2004;14(2):146–60.
62. Westen D, Novotny CM, Thompson-Brenner H. The empirical status of empirically supported psychotherapies: assumptions, findings, and reporting in controlled clinical trials. Psychol Bull 2004. https://doi.org/10.1037/0033-2909.130.4.631.
63. Wampold BE, Budge SL, Laska KM, et al. Evidence-based treatments for depression and anxiety versus treatment-as-usual: a meta-analysis of direct comparisons. Clin Psychol Rev 2011;31:1304–12.
64. Cuijpers P, Smit F, Bohlmeijer E, et al. Efficacy of cognitive-behavioural therapy and other psychological treatments for adult depression: meta-analytic study of publication bias. Br J Psychiatry 2010. https://doi.org/10.1192/bjp.bp.109.066001.
65. Shedler J. Where is the evidence for "evidence-based" therapy? Journal of Psychological Therapies in Primary Care 2015;4:47–59.
66. Driessen E, Van HL, Don FJ, et al. The efficacy of cognitive-behavioral therapy and psychodynamic therapy in the outpatient treatment of major depression: a randomized clinical trial. Am J Psychiatry 2013;170:1041–50.
67. Krueger RF. The structure of common mental disorders. Arch Gen Psychiatry 1999;56(10):921–6.
68. Brown TA, Chorpita BF, Barlow DH. Structural relationships among dimensions of the DSM-IV anxiety and mood disorders and dimensions of negative affect, positive affect, and autonomic arousal. J Abnorm Psychol 1998;107(2):179.
69. Watson D, Clark LA. Negative affectivity: the disposition to experience aversive emotional states. Psychol Bull 1984;96(3):465.
70. Barlow DH, Ellard KK, Sauer-Zavala S, et al. The origins of neuroticism. Perspect Psychol Sci 2014;9(5):481–96.
71. Krueger RF, McGue M, Iacono WG. The higher-order structure of common DSM mental disorders: internalization, externalization, and their connections to personality. Personal Individ Differ 2001;30(7):1245–59.
72. PDM Task Force. Psychodynamic diagnostic manual. Silver Spring (MD): Alliance of Psychoanalytic Organizations; 2006.
73. Bateman AW, Fonagy P. Handbook of mentalizing in mental health practice. London: APPI; 2011.
74. Wang PS, Berglund P, Olfson M, et al. Failure and delay in initial treatment contact after first onset of mental disorders in the National Comorbidity Survey Replication. Arch Gen Psychiatry 2005;62(6):603–13.
75. Wang PS, Lane M, Olfson M, et al. Twelve-month use of mental health services in the United States: results from the National Comorbidity Survey Replication. Arch Gen Psychiatry 2005;62(6):629–40.
76. Melek S, Norris D. Chronic conditions and comorbid psychological disorders. Seattle (WA): Milliman; 2008.
77. Luber MP, Hollenberg JP, Williams-Russo P, et al. Diagnosis, treatment, comorbidity, and resource utilization of depressed patients in a general medical practice. Int J Psychiatry Med 2000;30(1):1–14.
78. Deykin EY, Keane TM, Kaloupek D, et al. Posttraumatic stress disorder and the use of health services. Psychosom Med 2001;63(5):835–41.
79. US Department of Labor, Bureau of Labor Statistics. Employee tenure in 2016. Washington, DC: US Department of Labor Statistics; 2016.
80. Manning WG Jr, Wells KB, Duan N, et al. How cost sharing affects the use of ambulatory mental health services. JAMA 1986;256:1930–4.

81. Landerman L, Burns B, Swartz M, et al. The relationship between insurance coverage and psychiatric disorder in predicting use of mental health services. Am J Psychiatry 1994;151:1785–90.
82. Simon G, Grothaus L, Durham M, et al. Impact of visit copayments on outpatient mental health utilization by members of a health maintenance organization. Am J Psychiatry 1996;153:331–8.
83. Ravesteijn B, Schachar EB, Beekman ATF, et al. Association of cost sharing with mental health care use, involuntary commitment, and acute care. JAMA Psychiatry 2017;74(9):1–9.
84. Druss BG. Cost sharing and mental health care a cautionary tale from the Netherlands. JAMA Psychiatry 2017;74(9):940–1.
85. Lazar SG, editor. Psychotherapy is worth it: a comprehensive review of its cost effectiveness. Washington, DC: American Psychiatric Publishing; 2010.
86. Knoepflmacher D. Psychiatry and psychotherapy, 'medical necessity' in psychiatry: whose definition is it anyway? Psychiatric News 2016.
87. Substance Abuse and Mental Health Services Administration (SAMHSA). Medical necessity in private health plans implications for behavioral health care. Rockville (MD): Substance Abuse and Mental Health Services Administration; 2003.
88. Rosenbaum S, Kamoie B, Mauery DR, et al. Medical necessity in private health plans: implications for behavioral health care. DHHS Pub. No. (SMA) 03-3790. Rockville (MD): Center for Mental Health Services, Substance Abuse and Mental Health Services Administration; 2003.
89. Kessler S. Mental health parity: the patient protection and affordable care act and the parity definition implications. Hastings Sci Tech Law J 2014;6(2):145–66.
90. Field MJ, Lohr KN, editors. Clinical practice guidelines: directions for a new program. Institute of Medicine (US) Committee to Advise the Public Health Service on Clinical Practice Guidelines. Washington, DC: National Academies Press (US); 1990.
91. American Medical Association Statement to the Institute of Medicine's Committee on Determination of Essential Health Benefits, January 14, 2011.
92. American Psychiatric Association Official actions, position statement on medical necessity definition, 2015.
93. Mee-Lee D, Shulman GD, Fishman MJ, et al, editors. The ASAM criteria: treatment criteria for addictive, substance-related, and co-occurring conditions. 3rd edition. Carson City (NV): The Change Companies; 2013.
94. Merrick EL, Horgan CM, Garnick DW, et al. Accessing specialty behavioral health treatment in private health plans. J Behav Health Serv Res 2009;6(4):420–35.
95. Wickizer TM, Lessler D. Utilization management: issues, effects, and future prospects. Annu Rev Public Health 2002;23:233–54.

81. [illegible] MS, et al. The relationship between insurance coverage and psychiatric disorder in predicting use of mental health services. Am J Psychiatry 1994;151(12):1785-90.
82. Simon GE, Grothaus L, Durham ML, et al. Impact of visit copayments on outpatient mental health utilization by members of a health maintenance organization. Am J Psychiatry 1996;153(3):331-8.
83. Ravesteijn B, Schachar EB, Beekman ATF, et al. Association of cost sharing with mental health care use, involuntary commitment, and acute care. JAMA Psychiatry 2017;74(9):932-9.
84. Druss BG. Cost sharing and mental health care: a cautionary tale from the Netherlands. JAMA Psychiatry 2017;74(9):940.
85. Lazar SG, editor. Psychotherapy is worth it: a comprehensive review of its cost-effectiveness. Washington, DC: American Psychiatric Publishing; 2010.
86. Knoepflmacher D. Psychiatry and psychotherapy: medical necessity in psychotherapy, whose definition is it anyway? Psychiatric News 2016.
87. Substance Abuse and Mental Health Services Administration (SAMHSA). Medical necessity in private health plans: implications for behavioral health care. Rockville (MD): Substance Abuse and Mental Health Services Administration; 2003.
88. Rosenbaum S, Kamoie B, Mauery DR, et al. Medical necessity in private health plans: implications for behavioral health care. DHHS Pub. No. (SMA) 03-3790. Rockville (MD): Center for Mental Health Services, Substance Abuse and Mental Health Services Administration; 2003.
89. Kessler S. Mental health parity: the patient protection and affordable care act and the parity definition implications. Hastings Sci Tech Law J 2014;6(2):145-66.
90. Field MJ, Lohr KN, editors. Clinical practice guidelines: directions for a new program. Institute of Medicine (US) Committee to Advise the Public Health Service on Clinical Practice Guidelines. Washington, DC: National Academies Press; 1990.
91. American Medical Association Statement to the Institute of Medicine's Committee on Determination of Essential Health Benefits. January 14, 2011.
92. American Psychiatric Association Official actions. Position statement on medical necessity definition. 2015.
93. Mee-Lee D, Shulman GD, Fishman MJ, et al, editors. The ASAM criteria: treatment criteria for addictive, substance-related, and co-occurring conditions. 3rd edition. Carson City (NV): The Change Companies; 2013.
94. Merrick EL, Horgan CM, Garnick DW, et al. Accessing specialty behavioral health treatment in private health plans. J Behav Health Serv Res 2009;36(4):420-35.
95. Wickizer TM, Lessler D. Utilization management: issues, effects, and future prospects. Annu Rev Public Health 2002;23:233-54.

The Psychodynamic Treatment of Borderline Personality Disorder

An Introduction to Transference-Focused Psychotherapy

Barry L. Stern, PhD[a,*], Frank Yeomans, MD, PhD[b]

KEYWORDS

- Psychodynamic psychotherapy • Borderline personality disorder
- Exploratory psychotherapy • Transference

KEY POINTS

- The application of a twice-weekly exploratory psychotherapy, transference-focused psychotherapy (TFP), to patients with borderline personality disorder (BPD) is described in this article.
- The authors describe borderline personality as a psychopathology of internal object relations, and outline how TFP working with this internal structure, seeks to treat borderline psychopathology.
- An outline of the assessment and treatment protocol is described along with a case example to illustrate the same.

Borderline personality disorder (BPD) is a disorder characterized by instability in patients' sense of identity, as expressed in a stable representation of the self across situations and time and the ability to direct oneself in a consistent, deliberate, and productive manner in one's interpersonal and occupational functioning.[1] The difficulties in the realm of identity are accompanied by severe difficulties in regulation of emotions (intense anger, mood lability) and poor coping (impulsive, self-destructive behaviors). Patients' problematic experience of the self (identity) and poor emotion

Disclosure: The authors have no financial or commercial conflict of interest and the authors have not received any funding to directly support this work.
[a] Columbia University College of Physicians and Surgeons, Columbia University Center for Psychoanalytic Training and Research, 122 East 42nd Street, Suite 3200, New York, NY 10168, USA; [b] New York Presbyterian Hospital, Weill Medical College at Cornell University, 122 East 42nd Street, Suite 3200, New York, NY 10168, USA
* Corresponding author.
E-mail address: bs2137@cumc.columbia.edu

Psychiatr Clin N Am 41 (2018) 207–223
https://doi.org/10.1016/j.psc.2018.01.012
0193-953X/18/

regulation often play out on the stage of interpersonal relationships, which, for patients with borderline, are notoriously tumultuous.

The challenges for clinicians treating patients with borderline have long been recognized. Helping patients tolerate the intense feelings stimulated in them by the treatment situation and working to prevent the impulsive, often dangerous reactions to the same can be emotionally exhausting. Even when successful, the levels of frustration, concern, fear, and anger activated in us as therapists in response to our work with patients with borderline personality disorder can be difficult to bear.

The authors' task in this article is to provide an overview of how transference-focused psychotherapy (TFP),[2–4] a twice-weekly psychodynamic psychotherapy for BPD that is now being extended to other types of personality pathology,[5–7] conceptualizes, assesses, and treats borderline pathology. It is the intention of psychodynamically oriented clinicians, and TFP therapists in particular, to work at a level of depth that could yield structural change, that is, change in the psychological structures (identity, defensive style), that would in a meaningful and enduring way reshape the patients' experience of the self, subjectively and interpersonally, thus, more durably quieting the maladaptive traits and symptoms associated with borderline pathology. In addition to its effectiveness in reducing BPD symptoms, studies of TFP have indeed found it to be effective, in contrast to supportive psychodynamic therapy and Dialectical Behavior Therapy (DBT), in increasing reflective functioning[8] thought to be an indicator of structural change and in dimensions thought to constitute psychic structure as defined in the authors' model, that is, domains of identity and defensive functioning.[9]

TFP is the outgrowth of a group of clinicians and researchers working and studying over the past 30 years at the Personality Disorders Institute of the Weill Cornell Medical Center. Through weekly consultation and study group meetings, and multiple psychotherapy trials,[3,8,9] a conceptualization of the internal, underlying, psychological structural features of borderline pathology has been developed, along with an assessment method[10,11] and well-operationalized treatment protocol.[2,3] The work of TFP involves analyzing the defensive processes that support the split sense of self that is hypothesized to underlie many of the *Diagnostic and Statistical Manual of Mental Disorders'* (*DSM*) personality disorders, including BPD. The ultimate goal of TFP is to help patients better understand the need for and function of those defensive processes with the hope of promoting and helping patients to tolerate a more realistic, adaptive integration of positive and negative representations of self and others that will translate into a richer sense of self and a fuller appreciation of others; on the broadest level, the treatment helps individuals move from perceiving themselves and others through the lens of simple and extreme internal representations to appreciating their own and others' complexity.

BORDERLINE PERSONALITY ORGANIZATION AS A PATHOLOGY OF INTERNAL OBJECT RELATIONS

The authors' model of personality disorder, deriving from contemporary object relations theory, posits that experiences of the self in relation to others are organized in the developing mind according to a split between experiences that are rewarding, gratifying, and pleasurable and those that are frustrating and painful. Under conditions of adequate nurturance, stability, emotional containment, and within-normal-limits genetic loading, the developing child is eventually able to reach a stance in which important people in their world can be represented in a more realistic, balanced, and mixed representation, one in which the good qualities of the person are not lost to conscious awareness under conditions of stress or frustration (a whole-object position or object constancy). However, under adverse conditions (characterized by chronic trauma, parental abuse or neglect, a poor match between child temperament and parental attunement or empathic capacities, and/or a genetic loading for aggressive temperament), the frustrations presented to the child overwhelm the developing coping systems, resulting in a defensive split in the experience of the parental figures in which good experiences and representations of those figures are kept separate in the mind from bad/frustrating experiences and representations and with an overall emotional valence that is negative and tinged with aggression. Over time, these various experiences of the self-in-relation-to-other, whether good and bad representations are split or not, are consolidated or organized and internalized as a set of expectancies or relationship templates in the mind at which point they can be referred to as internal object relations or simply object relations.

The authors indeed think of these internal representations as *relations*, that is, a representation of the self, *linked by an affect*, to a representation of another (**Fig. 1**). Examples include, an inadequate self, linked by fear, to a critical other; a mistreated self, linked by rage, to an exploitive other; an accomplished self, linked by pride, to an admiring other. These relationships are *internal* relationships, all encoded in the psyche early in life through the impact of highly salient, patterned, *actual* relationships that, because of the impact of unconscious processes (desires, fears, fantasies), may take on an exaggerated nature as they are internalized in the psyche. In turn, these internal representations of relationships color and to some extent distort actual relationship experiences based on one's internal expectancies, wishes, and fears. It is the internal array of these self-object dyads, whether the positively and negatively valenced dyads are split or integrated, which are more prominent, regularly experienced, and affectively charged, that defines the quality of the individual's developing *identity*. Identity can be thought of as the ego function that organizes our internal object relations, in turn shaping both the structure (integrated, flexible vs split, rigid) and outward expression of the individual's personality as revealed to us in the consulting room.[11,12,13]

Identity pathology or diffusion is considered a hallmark of borderline disorders and is diagnosed when such a defensive split between good and bad internal representations or experiences of the self and others persists into adult life. Patients with BPD are characterized by black and white thinking, in which the self and others are experienced as caricatured extremes, with little nuance or integration of positive and negative attributes, and with rapid shifts between positive and negative experiences of self and others. This internal split leaves patients vulnerable to typical borderline symptoms, such as mood lability, idealization/devaluation, instability, and a lack of

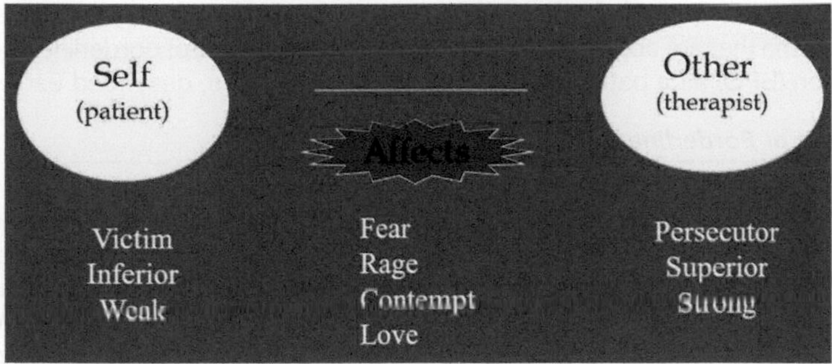

Fig. 1. The object relations dyad.

coherence in the sense of self, with corresponding difficulties in the steady, realistic experience of others.

Identity pathology is supported by patients' predominant use of what psychodynamic clinicians call splitting-based or primitive defenses. These defensive processes, which operate out of conscious awareness, serve to maintain the split between radically negative and positive experiences of the self and others that, were it to break down, would lead to affective experiences that would be disturbing or even overwhelming. Individuals with such split internal psychological organization do not generally consciously experience the aggressive, hostile affect within them as their own (even though they may express them in action). Aggressive affects are generally projected and seen as coming from others. This perception leads to a generally untrusting, even paranoid stance toward others, while protecting the self from the disturbing awareness that one's emotional difficulties emanate from within the self. Because of this, borderline patients often use the defense mechanism of omnipotent control. A strategy operating largely outside conscious awareness, in which the interpersonal dialogue and interaction with others are subtly or grossly controlled so as to bypass experiences or discussions that would be threatening to the self by challenging the patients' dominant narrative. This control operates so that the interpersonal dialogue and interaction bypass experiences or discussions that would be threatening to the self by challenging the patients' narrative version of how things are. Idealization/devaluation helps patients maintain the wished-for, all-good representations of the self or others, for example, but frequently results in sharp shifts to disappointments in self and others, thus, avoiding a more complicated, anxiety-laden but more realistic experience of self and others. Similarly, externalization helps patients maintain favorable images of the self, whereas projective identification results in the assignment (and often unconscious induction) of unwanted self-representations to others, with the patients still expressing (identifying with) those very characteristics, albeit unconsciously.

It is likely that many of the problems that characterize the personality disorder diagnostic system in the latest iterations of the *DSM* (eg, criterion overlap, heterogeneity within diagnostic categories)[14,15] can be explained, in part, by the hypothesis that most personality disorders share underlying features that have yet to be fully elaborated and incorporated into the diagnostic system. The *DSM* in versions IV and 5 suggest this very fact in the narrative introduction to the personality disorders, noting that the personality disorders as a group are defined by some combination of problems in self-regulation, the experience of self and others, and corresponding interpersonal difficulties. The Alternative Model for the assessment of personality disorders in *DSM 5* elaborates these criteria even further. In combination with several maladaptive personality traits that vary across the various personality disorders, the general criteria specify impairment in self and interpersonal functioning, defined further as difficulties in the areas of identity and self-direction (self) and empathy and intimacy (interpersonal relations), criteria that are congruent with the Kernberg's concept of borderline personality organization (BPO) as a pathology of internal object relations, described earlier.[12,13]

Assessment of Borderline Personality Organization

A careful evaluation typically extending across 2 initial meetings is central to the initiation of TFP. The evaluation sessions are directed by the therapist, allowing him or her to obtain the information necessary for establishing both phenomenological (*DSM*) and structural diagnoses and identifying borderline features, such as impulsivity or self-injury/suicidality, that might complicate or threaten the nature of the treatment being proposed. During the evaluation session, the TFP-trained therapist typically follows the outline of the structural interview, a free-form clinical interview that asks the patients to describe current areas of difficulty (emotional, physical, and cognitive) with the therapist listening and probing the nature, extent, and history of those difficulties.[12] While establishing the presence or absence of axis I pathology, the therapist is also taking note of the patients' behavior during the interview and defensive style in response to the interviewer's questions: are patients guarded, defensive, and hostile or are the patients' responses believable, elaborated, and realistic, clarifying openly issues that may have been at first unclear? And what is the interviewer's feeling during the interview: are his or her probes welcome and considered or are they dismissed, with him or her feeling devalued, stonewalled, and controlled? The concurrent test of the defensive system through gentle bids for elaboration and from the presentation of conflicting pieces of information in the patients' narrative that make the presentation unclear, points either toward or away from a diagnosis of splitting as a predominant defensive strategy.

The diagnosis of BPO is further clarified through the therapist's direct inquiry related to the patients' sense of identity, his or her sense of coherence and authenticity across time and situations, the narrative description of self (elaborated, multifaceted, nuanced vs superficial, caricatured, stilted), and the sense of stability of moods and self-esteem over time. The patients' ability to direct themselves in the area of the primary role (work/school), the capacity to invest the self in these areas as well as in recreational pursuits, is also diagnostic of identity health or pathology.[a]

Direct assessment of features of BPD, including mood lability and a propensity toward anger and impulsivity, including self-injury and suicidality, is also required in order to establish the specific personality disorder diagnosis. Assessment of stability and valence of self-esteem, feelings of entitlement, the capacity for empathy, the experience of envy, and the patients' need for and response to admiration and its absence would help to clarify the presence of significant narcissistic features within the borderline range. Within the borderline range, 3 specific factors help locate patients on a spectrum of severity and provide a guideline for prognosis:

- What is the nature of the patients' aggression? How controlled, severe, and frequent is their expressed aggression; is it directed against the self, others, or both?
- What is the patients' capacity for guilt, remorse, concern for their actions, and the effects of the same on others? Are patients guided by any internal moral compass that can serve as a check against impulsive, reactive aggression?
- What is the state of the patients' interpersonal relationships? Are patients socially connected, are there social supports, and do patients have any nonexploitive, reciprocal relationships with others?

The greater the extent of the aggression, as described earlier, the less concern and remorse related to that aggression; the poorer the state of the patients' interpersonal relationships, the lower in the BPO spectrum the patients fall and the poorer the patients' prognosis in TFP.

After confirming the diagnosis, 2 further crucial steps are required to complete the pretreatment process. First, the patients' *DSM* diagnosis, and the syndrome of BPO, the structural diagnosis, must be shared with patients. Although controversial, the

[a] The Structured Interview of Personality Organization, a semistructured interview that operationalizes the aforementioned structural interview, provides clear language for the assessment of identity, primitive defenses, and several additional domains relevant to the assessment of personality organization.[11]

authors often find that sharing this diagnosis, and explaining the patients' symptoms as reflecting an inner problem with one's sense of self (identity), with corresponding difficulties in self-regulation and emotion regulation, and difficulties in interpersonal relationships, helps patients to contextualize the PD symptoms in the story of the person. Said differently, that one's underlying difficulties feeling at home in oneself, stable in one's sense of self over time, with corresponding shifts in the experience of self and others, helps to explain the symptoms of BPD as well as the related feelings of emptiness, depression, and anxiety that often bring patients into treatment in the first place.

Second, and the last step before initiating TFP proper, is the establishment of a *treatment contract*, an agreement with patients as to the conditions of treatment, the mutual expectations of the therapist and patients, and an agreement concerning the management of patients' behaviors that have the potential to disrupt the conduct of an exploratory, psychodynamic treatment.[16] For patients prone to self-injury, medication misuse or alcohol/drug abuse, eating disordered behavior, or excessive out-of-session contact with the therapist, these behaviors can at times pose a serious threat to the patients' well-being and also to the treatment and, if uncontrolled, can compromise the therapist's ability to work with patients from the exploratory stance required to conduct TFP. Participation in adjunctive treatment groups related to alcohol or drug abuse or eating disorders or merely an agreement to refrain from and promptly report and seek treatment of self-injury when it does occur are examples of parameters that provide both the patients and therapist some reassurance that the treatment can proceed without these issues compromising either's ability to participate in the treatment. Adherence to the treatment contract is often inconsistent in the treatment of patients with BPD, and instances of a lack of adherence would be explored in the therapy; but without establishing such parameters at the outset, the treatment cannot become the sufficiently bounded and containing venue for the discussion and analysis of the patients' inner conflicts and lived difficulties (for further elucidation of issues related to treatment contracting see [2,16]). An additional aspect of the treatment contract involves a stipulation that patients engage in some structured activity (job, education, training) during the course of treatment. This stipulation guards against the treatment supporting secondary gain of the illness in the form of passive, or exploitative, retreat from the responsibilities of living. This aspect of the treatment contract also forces patients to confront the actual capacities for functioning, as well as their limitations, to engage in real-time conflicts related to submission and collaboration, ambition, striving, and the associated impulse to withdraw from life's challenges.

In addition to these patient-specific parameters, the universal features of TFP treatments (the twice-weekly frequency, clearly establishing that the treatment takes place in person during the sessions, and limiting extra session contact to logistical matters, ie, issues related to vacations, scheduling, and billing) are also clarified. Establishing these aspects at the start of treatment allows the therapist and patients the ability to explore deviations, or expressed wishes to deviate from the contract (and the meaning of the same), and what they say about the patients' personality as it gets played out in the relationship between patients and therapist in the treatment process.

CASE OVERVIEW

When Tina presented to the therapist, self-referred, for the treatment of her BPD, the therapist was somewhat taken aback. "I found you on the web, and need an expert in borderline; I know I can't afford you, but I'll get a job to pay for the treatment because I know I'll die if I can't get help for this." She was self-educated about her condition, spot-on in her self-diagnosis, and indeed serious in her desire for treatment. Tina had been through various treatments for depression and anxiety, none of which had addressed her outbursts of rage, her impulsive suicidality, the volatile social and romantic relationships that she had burned through, and the toxic attachment to what seemed to be a bipolar and highly abusive mother, with whom she was currently living.

Tall and attractive, Tina glided down the halls of the therapist's suite and fell into the office chair, immediately dropping her head dramatically onto the armrest and flipping her long hair over her face. From this awkward physical perch, in the most childlike voice imaginable, she articulated her self experience: "Nobody loves me. I feel like a mishmash of broken parts that nobody else wants." She described never feeling sufficiently attended to, from periods of severe and traumatic early childhood neglect to her current life when she could never obtain sufficient attention or praise from those close to her along with associated outbursts of rage when she experienced insufficient regard or attention. She described the experience of feeling repeatedly let down, taken advantage of, and mistreated, a victim, in her mind, of a callous, cruel world. Collateral reports from the hospital from which she had recently been discharged (after being hospitalized for 2 weeks after a suicide gesture) indicated that she had spat on the admitting nurse and had several outbursts of rage while on the unit, with little demonstration of remorse. Tina dismissed these incidents, still in her most high-pitched, childish voice, as completely justified and in no way contradicting her sense of self as a victim. She became silent and angry with the therapist when pressed further on this contradiction, which suggested the operation of splitting-based defenses that serve to reinstate in her mind the internal situation with herself as the helpless victim of a cruel, persecutory outside world while elucidating that very same dyad, for the first time, in the transference.[b]

Tina had graduated college but with tremendous difficulty, including 2 leaves of absence due to depression. The therapist's inquiry into these episodes yielded a vague report that did not confirm the presence of a major affective illness. Rather, both involved lengthy stories of interpersonal drama and conflict, one involving her mother and the other involving the breakup of a chaotic long-term relationship. Tina's history of alcohol abuse and cutting were explored and, again, seem to be related to the volatility of her interpersonal relationships. Rage at the hint of abandonment by boyfriends, impulsive coping with interpersonal stressors, associated with rage and mood lability, all suggested a borderline diagnosis. Tina's experience of the self alternated sharply, with her enacting rage and control while alternately feeling weak and victimized. Her tastes and preferences shifted according to whom she was with as did her dress and her expression of her values (*very* strongly held but at the same time regularly shifting). Her self-esteem vacillated between her feeling broken and incompetent and a realistic appraisal of her actual talent and intellect; Tina had in fact begun studies at a prestigious law school only to drop out late in her first term under the stress and volatility associated with a new romantic relationship.

Tina's prognosis was guarded; severe hostility and aggression were typical, somewhat uncontrolled, and expressed without apparent concern for their effects on

---

[b] In the case of patients operating under the influence of splitting-based defenses, the therapist's bid to have patients clarify conflicting pieces of data (between either 2 aspects of a verbal report, perhaps been 2 informants, or between the patients' verbal report and behavior outside the session) often results in a more paranoid stance and in the enactment of the internal world *in the transference*. Once in the transference, it can be explored from an emotionally active stance in the very moment when it is being experienced, a feature of the treatment process that is central to TFP.

others. Tina's interpersonal relationships were chaotic, on and off, and unsatisfying; she had almost no true social and emotional supports. Tina's work ethic, intelligence, and the absence of antisocial features, however, suggested the potential for growth in TFP. Tina agreed to a treatment contract in which she would refrain from cutting herself or from other self-injury, agreeing that she would contact an emergency department or call 911 if she experienced urges that she could not control to hurt herself in such a manner. She agreed to adjunctive Alcoholics Anonymous meetings if she continued to engage in binge-drinking episodes and also agreed to seek employment. And indeed, shortly after the start of treatment, Tina found a job as a paralegal, which she sustained throughout our work, and at which she excelled.

THE PRACTICE OF TRANSFERENCE-FOCUSED PSYCHOTHERAPY

The work of TFP involves setting up a therapeutic environment in which the patients' split-off, internalized object relations (ones that are subjectively experienced by patients and ones that are enacted in behavior or experienced via projection by those in the patients' surround) are reenacted and observed in the treatment relationship. The conditions of treatment include elements such as session frequency, the instruction to the patients to engage in a modified free-associative style with particular attention to priorities related to self-destructive and treatment-interfering behaviors, and the therapist's stance, which is limited to efforts to clarify, challenge, and explicate through interpretation rather than providing overt guidance and support. All of these elements are designed to facilitate the reactivation of the patients' internal object relations in the treatment, where they can be explored, interpreted, and discussed.

The authors' summary of TFP as a treatment involves a description of 3 elements (**Fig. 2**). The authors refer to strategies in TFP as the long-term goals over the course of treatment, their efforts to help patients make sense of their inner world of object relations, the associated emotional states, and to track the manifestations of the same in their daily interpersonal life and in the treatment relationship. The tactics of TFP establish the boundaries and priorities of the therapeutic process, much of

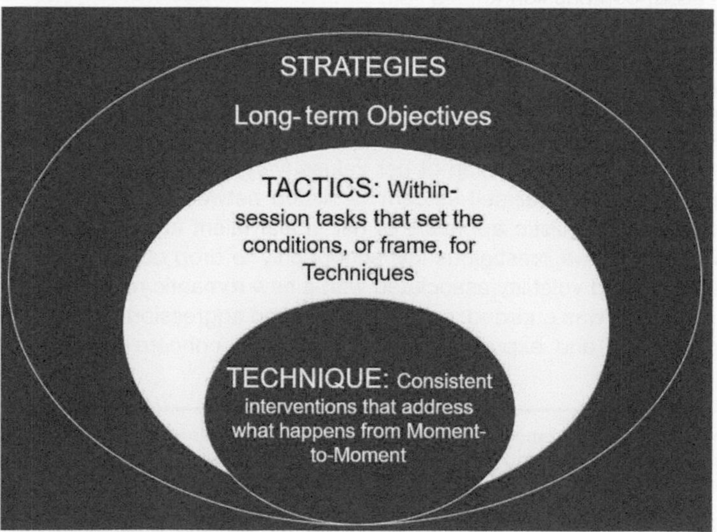

Fig. 2. The relationship of strategies, tactics, and techniques.

what clinicians mean when speaking of the treatment frame. Last, the techniques of TFP are the interventions that the authors practice within the sessions, including the nuances of their interpretive technique, the stance from which they interpret, and the data they use to inform their interpretations. All 3 of these aspects are discussed in turn, below.

The authors' discussion of the strategies, tactics, and techniques of TFP takes place through the lens of the treatment of Tina. The initial several months of treatment were marked by Tina's presentation of the chaos and emotional volatility of her life. Anger at her mother's verbal abuse, which in turn amplified an internal sense of being unworthy of love, stupid, and unable to make good life choices. Tina tested the treatment contract, calling the therapist provocatively one evening, drunk after a fight with a man she had been seeing, unclear if she could keep herself safe or not (The therapist was able to speak with a friend who agreed in this instance to get her home safely, which in fact occurred.) Their discussions of such incidents and of her rage at others and at the therapist dominated their early work, with Tina experiencing the therapist in 2 ways: as a cold, uncaring, neglectful parent, with her a victim of the therapist's neglect and as an idealized savior who, if she could only get the therapist to, would love her and make all her difficulties and conflicts go away.

STRATEGIES

Every mode of treatment must answer the following question: For what do we listen in the treatment and where and when do we choose to intervene? In TFP, within a session and over time, therapeutic attention is constantly tracking the dominant affect at any given moment. Are patients angry, sad, contemptuous, arrogant, for example, and how is the affect being expressed? One consistent observation from the authors' work with patients with BPD is that often the most important information at any given moment is being conveyed less through the patients' verbal narrative than through the patients' behavior, or via projection, experienced in the countertransference. Indeed, the therapist's reflection on his or her own affect at any point (why am I feeling unsettled, confused, compassionate, loving, rageful?) can be very helpful identifying the dominant affect.

Once the dominant affect is identified, we can begin to attach to it the patients' self-representation that is active at that moment and the corresponding representation of the therapist. It is this basic framework, described visually in **Fig. 1**, that is the primary compass for intervention in TFP. The first task is to name the actors and the interaction or to share with patients how they seem to be experiencing themselves and the therapist, as the affects shift across the session, and to ask questions (clarifications) that help to better understand both the affects and self states active in those moments. Helping patients learn to track their affective states and how they are feeling about themselves and the therapist at those moments is the baseline work of TFP. What the authors often find in patients whose internal world is unintegrated as described earlier is that they experience abrupt shifts in their self-other experience, that is, that the roles, or poles of the dyad reflected in **Fig. 1**, reverse: At one moment the patients feel weak, inferior, and are fearful (the dominant affect in patients) of attack. Yet, in response to an intervention inviting the patients to reflect on something painful, or to attempt to clarify something confusing to the therapist, or perhaps in absence of some expected validation or support, the patients may move suddenly to the attack, berating the therapist (**Fig. 3**). Such reversals in the dominant self-object dyad can also happen unprompted by the therapist: in one session a patient

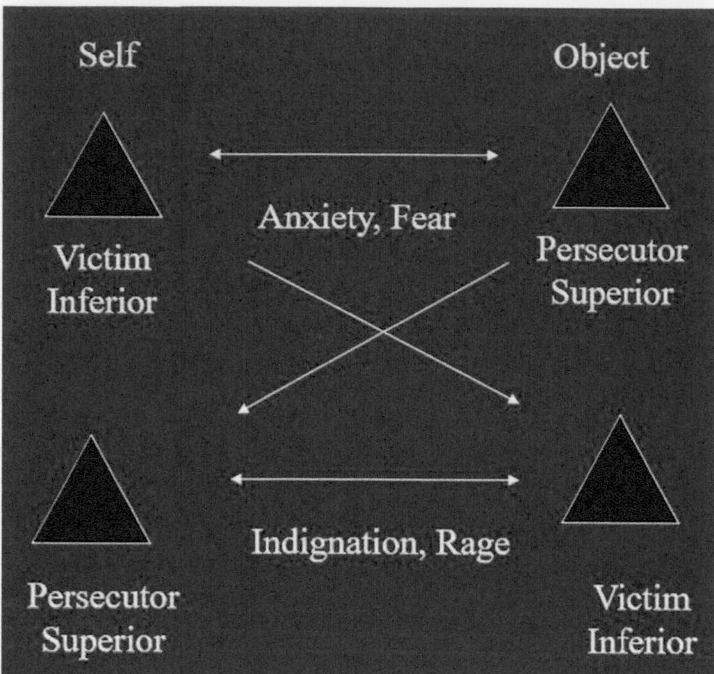

Fig. 3. Oscillation of the object relations dyad. The identification is with the entire relationship not just with the self-representation or the object representation. The dyad exists within the individual; its basic impact is on the self relating to self, although it regularly gets expressed between self and others.

arrives feeling downtrodden, ineffective, weak, and envious of those whom she sees as more comfortable, healthy, attractive, or successful; another time the patient may come in full of indignant rage, contemptuous and superior, of others and the therapist. Part of the strategies of TFP is to track these shifts, or oscillations in the self-object dyads as they unfold in the treatment process.

Although much of the work with the authors' patients in the borderline range is dominated by the work with their patients' negative affects, their anger, contempt, disappointment, and frustration. In TFP, the authors always strive to bear in mind that these persecutory dyads generally defend against awareness of a set of wished-for relationships in which an idealized self is met by and cared for by an idealized world and therapist/caretaker. The authors' experience with patients in the borderline range, however, is that these ideal wished-for relationship dyads are also fraught, because they, like the negative persecutory dyads, do not fit the complexity of the real world. Because the internal world is managed through splitting-based defenses, the wished-for relationship is not simply a realistic good enough other but an idealized other, one that is unrealistic in that it never disappoints, frustrates, or deprives. The following might be the expression of an idealized dyad: I want to be your perfect patient, saying the right things, deserving of praise and affection, and I long for your perfect, never-wavering attention and care.

Although patients might on the surface deny this wish as unrealistic, their difficulty tolerating a view of the self that could be kind and smart but at times demanding, angry, and confused generates a pressure for perfection in the self and a corresponding need for perfection in the therapist, constituting an idealized dyad that superficially feels positively valenced but that also screens considerable aggression, an aggression that inevitably arises with the frustration of not finding the other, as ideal as hoped (or, alternately, not being the ideal self). When the brittle, idealized bubble bursts in the process, the shift is often abrupt, throwing the patient and therapist right back into the persecutory sphere: I was no longer the therapist from whom you wanted care (because I presumably have something of value that you need); I am now a depriving sadist who never understands you and endlessly frustrates you because I do not provide perfect care.

In this manner, the authors think in TFP of the layering of dyads (**Fig. 4**). Persecutory dyads can often shield (underneath the surface level fear and anger) a powerfully longed-for relationship that patients can hardly bear to express. This situation is frequently the case with narcissistic patients for whom the admission of any desire for something or someone not part of or fully possessed or controlled by the self would be a humiliating admission of dependency and need.[7,17,18] Analysis of the idealized dyad, along with the implicit intolerance of *any* imperfection in self or therapist/other, and of the relationship between the idealized and persecutory sphere is the last and most far-reaching level of the longer-term TFP strategies and the level that ultimately contributes to the easing of the rigid splitting of positive and negative sectors of experience that characterize the internal world of patients in the borderline range.

TACTICS

The tactics of TFP involve the establishment of conditions for psychodynamic treatment that will allow for the safe and effective conduct of TFP, that is, the exploration and containment of the urgent priorities and clinical difficulties in the patients' life, in a format that the authors have outlined as effective for borderline pathology. As discussed earlier, the treatment contract establishes the logistical frame of the treatment as well as patient-specific conditions designed to limit self-destructive acting out so as to protect both patient and therapist, and their abiltity together to conduct TFP. Other tactics in TFP involve the patients' adherence to the treatment priorities, in which free association is modified to reflect a prioritization of self-destructive or

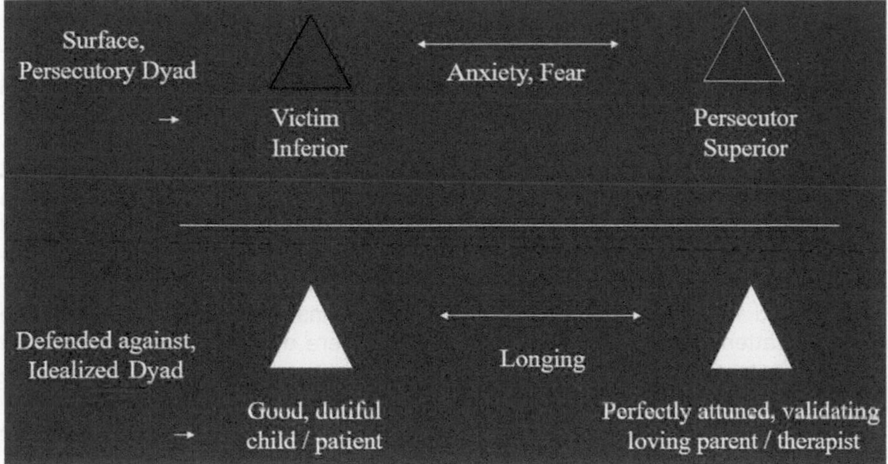

Fig. 4. Layering object relations dyads.

suicidal impulses, followed by behaviors that might interfere with the treatment (urges to skip sessions, quit, change medications, make major life changes, and so forth) followed by any other material that reflects the central conflicts and difficulties in the patients' life and for which they sought treatment. The aforementioned tactics, and the central guideline for the therapist's listening stance of tracking and intervening around the area of the dominant affect, is a final within-session tactic in TFP.

TECHNIQUES

TFP therapists strive to intervene with their patients from a stance of *technical neutrality*. Such a listening and interpretive stance does not imply indifference or a lack of affective engagement but rather one in which the therapists' affective responses are used to inform them as to the dominant self-object dyad, and their interventions remain focused on elucidating and interpreting, rather than taking one particular side in the patients' conflicts or promoting one part of themselves in contradiction to another. In fact, a key difference between TFP and more supportive-expressive psychodynamic techniques[19] is that in TFP therapists do not see their role as one of actively promoting the healthier, more likable or socially desirable parts of the patients. Rather, their task is help patients see the complexity of their selves and others and understand their difficulty retaining and living with that complexity and the need for the defensive processes used to keep unwanted experiences of self and others separate. Technical neutrality is not a pure state that can be objectively discerned. Our own internal pressures, desires, and limitations pull us in one direction or another with respect to patients' conflicts. And for sure our patients would, in many cases, love for us to tell them what to do and whom to love and to play the role of the guru. Part of our therapeutic awareness in TFP involves attending to neutrality, thinking about why we have deviated, and how to return to a more neutral stance. In certain cases, say involving dangerous acting out, we need to move out of neutrality deliberately and authoritatively to protect the patient or the treatment. Such deviations are to be expected. Once the crisis is averted, however, a discussion with patients of the conditions that drew the therapist into such a supportive or directive role should ensue.

The technique of *transference analysis* is used throughout the process of TFP. In tracking affects that emerge in the treatment process, and through our interventions, we invariably witness the reactivation of patients' internal object relations as experienced in the patient-therapist dyad. We see a dominant self-object representation say, in the case of Tina, figuring herself as a weak victim, needing the therapist's care and of the therapist figured as dismissive, mean, and insufficiently attentive. The identification of the dyad active at any given moment in the patient-therapist relationship (see **Fig. 1**), and the dominant affect in the patients associated with the self-representation, and the dominant affect associated with what is projected by the patients, that is, the countertransference, is the main thinking activity of the therapist in TFP.

Associated with the consistent attention to and analysis of transference is the therapists' attention to their *countertransference*, here defined as reactions to the patients in total, but particularly in response to the patients' transference, their projection into to the therapist of unwanted, difficult-to-tolerate self states and representations. It is well known that patients in the borderline range, because of the intensity of affects and the predominance of projection-based defenses, pose significant countertransference challenges to therapists. We feel pressured to be the good object, sensing our patients' needs and/or fearing our patients' anger, and can easily be seduced by their loving and erotic feelings (sometimes more a manifestation of their aggression or devaluation than love) and repelled by their shamelessness and callous disregard for self and others. Awareness and tolerance of one's countertransference and the capacity to contain one's own intense affects are central features of countertransference management and also central to our ability to intervene from a technically neutral position.

The primary technique of TFP involves the interpretive process,[2,3,20] one that closely tracks the strategies of TFP outlined earlier, that is, identifying and naming the dyads as they emerge, their oscillation in the treatment process, and their defensive function against other layers of dyads. *Clarification* involves efforts to understand with the patients what dyad is dominant at a given moment, to *seek* clarification as to what the patients are telling us at a given moment and why, and how they feel about what they are saying. Our clarifications help us to identify the dyad, for example, with Tina, her sense of self as a weak victim, needing the therapist's care, and of the therapist figured as dismissive, mean, and insufficiently attentive. *Confrontation* should not be confrontational or adversarial but rather involves the tactful presentation of contradictory aspects of the patients' experience to then, for examination: You say you're so afraid, yet you are scowling, in a manner one might take to be threatening. You're speaking about an event you said was extremely painful, yet your expression seems to have a wry smile, as though you were almost playfully curious about what my reaction will be. Confrontations, which are essentially an invitation to reflect, can be difficult for patients, as they serve as the gateway technique for the analysis of splitting; through confrontation we effectively point to different parts of patients that are being kept separate from one another. Confrontations are also central to the second level of interpretation and strategy in TFP wherein we work with the rapid reversal of the dominant surface dyads (see **Fig. 3**).

	Have you noticed, Tina, that in most sessions, you start off in this very quiet, meek voice, as though you're this lost child needing someone to take care of her?
Tina	(childlike, pouty, but with a smile) Why are you picking on me?
	I'm struck here: you navigated college and did well, and are now doing sophisticated legal work at a high level of skill and organization - seems hard to reconcile that with the little girl you present to me.
Tina	That's different. That's there, at work. That's not how I really am.
	Really are, or is it that there are two parts that are both really you, but that it's hard to show me both sides. Here, I have to be the strong/competent one, and you the one needing the attention and care.
Tina	I've never been taken care of; nobody cares to pay attention to me.
	So I wonder if that's the point: if seeing me as competent and you as the weak one needing care keeps you from avoiding the anxiety of being competent yourself. If you're competent, I imagine you feel anxious you might lose the attention and care that you for so long have been fixated on.

In this example, the therapist works to present to Tina a contradiction between her verbal report and behavior in session and information from elsewhere in her life, offering a trial interpretation related to her need to keep these parts of herself separate.

This dyad was just one of the dominant dyads that Tina presented in the authors' work. Early in the treatment, they also began to explore the vicissitudes of the dismissing, cruel parts of herself previously projected into and experienced in the person of the therapist, now enacted at various points by Tina herself. The task was to help Tina become aware, through tracking these oscillations, that both of these poles belonged to *her*. Tina was highly argumentative, ironic for someone overtly demanding greater attention and care, frequently rejecting the therapist's observations, finding them difficult to tolerate and in turn dismissing the therapist. Over the initial months of the treatment, Tina would at times present in a state of disappointment or contempt for the therapist and the treatment, for example, "This isn't helping, what are we even talking about anyway, how is *this* supposed to help me?" In these moments, the therapist had access to a part of Tina that could be cold, unforgiving, and dismissive, with the therapist in the role of passive victim to her attacks, representations quite at odds with her dominant experience. The task here is both to acknowledge the shift in roles and to propose a hypothesis as what might motivate both the shift and necessitate the more polarized experience of self and other. This segment followed Tina's discussion of an annoyance related to her work and a brief mutual pause of several seconds in which the therapist was contemplating privately what she had shared.

Tina	You're not saying anything. Well this really is helpful (sarcasm).
Th	Tell me more about what was going on in your mind during my silence?
Tina	In my mind? I'm thinking great. You never give me anything. I tell you I'm upset about this work situation and you're silent. All I want to do is feel better, and that's what I come to you for, and you tell me all these bad things about myself or you're silent.
Th	You're anticipating I'm going to disappoint or be critical of you, that it won't be enough, that I...
Tina	You got it right for once! Bravo. Yes, you give me nothing. NOTHING.
Th	You seem more bent on telling me what I'm not giving you, what I'm going to do or not do, much more than actually *listening* to anything I might have to say. (Playfully now) You're giving *me* nothing now, in terms of *your* attention, and now I'm rejected.
Tina	Ha ha...nice move (pause)
Th	Nice as in manipulative....or nice as in *maybe something to look at here*? You can get into a mode with me at times where you need to insist on my uselessness, are not open to anything I might have to offer. You become the rejecting one: fair?
Tina	A bit.
Th	It seems that you look to me anticipating that I'll be cruel and rejecting, leaving you with nothing. To see *yourself* as the one who can also be rejecting is overwhelming, you feel then like *you* are the bad one. And I wonder if that leads to the uncomfortable question of whether people might actually have things to offer you, that you have a hard time accepting.

Tracking these shifts or oscillations within the persecutory sphere was central in expanding Tina's understanding of the link between various parts of her self and her emotional states and helping her form a more balanced and full appreciation of herself. It is only at this point, when patients can reclaim some aspects of the self previously managed through projection, that patients can begin to see the self and others with increased complexity rather than in the exaggerated ways that reflect the distortions of self and others affected by projection and other splitting-based mechanisms.

Although the aforementioned excerpt focused on oscillation of the dyad within the persecutory sphere, note also the hint of the idealizing dyad: "All I want is to feel better...." This point provides a useful transition to the third level of interpretation in TFP and the third aspect of the treatment strategies discussed earlier, namely, the interpretation of the layering of dyads.

Tina	Ok, so I'm dismissive. Now what? (pause) Sometimes your silence...I just don't know what to do with it. I feel like you're just leaving the problem with me.
Th	Your sarcasm around that, earlier, was biting: you are so ready for me to fail you.
Tina	This doesn't feel good. I don't leave here feeling better.
Th	You sought this treatment out from the part of you that knows that I'm not some therapy guru or emotional surgeon... no ability here to extract those bad feelings fully...
Tina	Of course I know that.
Th	And I know you do...Yet it seems that you also come in here with a different part of you active: the compliant, dutiful patient, expecting a response from me that is fully validating and that will somehow eradicate all the bad feelings you are sitting with, uncertainty, insecurity, your sense of being alone in the world, your impatience and frustration... and when I hesitate or pause, and you expect I'm going to fail you...
Tina	IT DOESN'T HELP ME OUTSIDE OF HERE, when I feel this way
Th	And then I'm nothing: the therapist you wanted something important from 2 minutes ago, who can really, really help you, becomes totally useless, depriving and cruel.
Tina	It feels that way.
Th	So hard to hold both experiences of me in mind: someone from whom you want something important, even if it leaves you with some difficult feelings and work to do. Holding onto an experience of me as both giving yet frustrating, caring yet at times disagreeing with you, is so difficult and threatening. The feeling is that what you need so much is compromised, *totally*, if I can't take care of everything, perfectly.

Tina would often portray herself as an attentive, compliant, and dutiful patient (child); she paid her bill regularly, got a job as discussed in the initial meetings, promptly, and said proudly how she had incorporated things they had discussed in their work. This experience of herself in the treatment paralleled her desire to be a dutiful, attentive daughter, friend, and girlfriend. And this representation of an all-good, dutiful self was accompanied by her longing for a fully receptive, admiring, and validating other (therapist, parent, friend, and so forth). The only flaw in this model is its failure to account for human fallibilty, that is, reality. The therapist's failure to understand her quickly enough, seeing things that felt important but of which she seemed unaware, and, above all, the fact that the therapist's best work would still not fully resolve her difficulties, leaving her with some painful feelings and difficult choices, was at times utterly intolerable. At such moments, the brittle idealized dyad would abruptly shatter and the dominant object-relation would become reinstated, with the therapist being cruel, dismissive, and useless.

Segments such as these, repeated over time and across various sets of dyads, ultimately help to break down the rigid split between idealized and persecutory segments of relationship experiences, leading to their integration, the resolution of identity diffusion as primitive defenses start to relax, and the corresponding ability to better modulate the intense affect states that characterize our patients' lives. That is, the brittle hypomanic, euphoric states become more integrated with other periods associated with persecutory, hostile, dysphoric states.

The authors hope that this overview of TFP and the case illustrating TFP with Tina has helped provide a lively and realistic sense of how this modified psychoanalytic treatment, specifically tailored to the pathology of split internal object relations, can be helpful in the treatment of borderline pathology. As a group, the authors continue to work to refine their theory and technique, particularly in response to developing empirical work on borderline pathology and their psychotherapeutic study of patients with personality disorder.

REFERENCES

1. American Psychiatric Association. Diagnostic and statistical manual of mental disorders. 5th edition. Arlington (VA): American Psychiatric Publishing; 2013.
2. Yeomans FE, Clarkin JF, Kernberg OF. Transference-focused psychotherapy for borderline personality disorder: a clinical guide. Washington, DC: American Psychiatric Publishing; 2015.
3. Clarkin JF, Yeomans FE, Kernberg OF. Psychotherapy for borderline patients: an object relations approach. Washington, DC: American Psychiatric Press; 2006.
4. Clarkin JF, Levy KN, Lenzenweger MF, et al. Evaluating three treatments for borderline personality disorder: a multiwave study. Am J Psychiatry 2007; 164(6):922–8.
5. Caligor E, Kernberg OF, Clarkin J. Handbook of dynamic psychotherapy for higher-level personality. Washington, DC: American Psychiatric Publishing; 2007.
6. Hersh R, Caligor E, Yeomans F. Fundamentals of transference-focused psychotherapy: application in psychiatric and medical settings. Cham, Switzerland: Springer Nature; 2017.
7. Stern BL, Diamond D, Yeomans FE. Transference-focused psychotherapy for narcissistic personality disorder: engaging patients in the early treatment process. Psychoanalytic Psychol 2017;34(4):381–96.
8. Levy K, Meehan KB, Kelly KM, et al. Change in attachment patterns and reflective function in a randomized control trial of transference-focused psychotherapy for borderline personality disorder. J Consult Clin Psychol 2006;74:1027–40.
9. Doering S, Hörz S, Rentrop M, et al. Transference-focused psychotherapy v. treatment by community psychotherapists for borderline personality disorder: randomized controlled trial. Br J Psychiatry 2010;196(5):389–95.
10. Lenzenweger MF, Clarkin JF, Kernberg OF, et al. The inventory of personality organization: psychometric properties, factorial composition, and criterion relations with affect, aggressive dyscontrol, psychosis proneness, and self-domains in a nonclinical sample. Psychol Asst 2001;13:577–91.
11. Stern B, Caligor E, Clarkin JF, et al. The Structured Interview of Personality Organization (STIPO): preliminary psychometrics in a clinical sample. J Pers Assess 2010;92:35–44.
12. Kernberg OF. Severe personality disorders. New Haven (CT): Yale; 1984.
13. Kernberg OF, Caligor E. A psychoanalytic theory of personality disorders. In: Lenzenweger M, Clarkin J, editors. Major theories of personality disorder. New York: Guilford; 2005.
14. Westen D, Arkowitz-Westen L. Limitations of axis II in diagnosing personality pathology in clinical practice. Am J Psychi 1998;155:1767–71.
15. Verheul R. Clinical utility of dimensional models for personality pathology. In: Widiger TA, Simonsen E, Sirovatka PJ, et al, editors. Dimensional models of personality disorders: refining the research agenda for DSM-V. Washington, DC: American Psychiatric Association; 2006. p. 203–18.
16. Yeomans FE, Delaney J, Levy K. Behavior action in TFP: the role of the treatment contract in transference-focused psychotherapy. Psychotherapy 2017;54(3): 260–6.
17. Caligor E, Levy K, Yeomans FE. Narcissistic personality disorder: diagnostic and clinical challenges. Am J Psychi 2015;172:415–22.
18. Kernberg OF. An overview of the treatment of severe narcissistic pathology. Int J Psychoanal 2014;95(5):865–88.

19. Rockland LH. Supportive therapy for borderline patients: a psychodynamic approach. New York: Guilford; 1992.
20. Caligor E, Diamond D, Yeomans FE, et al. The interpretive process in psychoanalytic psychotherapy of borderline pathology. J Am Psychoanalytic Assoc 2009; 52(2):271–301.

A Psychodynamic Approach for the General Psychiatrist

Using Transference-Focused Psychotherapy Principles in Acute Care Settings

Richard G. Hersh, MD*

KEYWORDS

• Personality disorders • Transference • Psychodynamic psychotherapy
• General psychiatry • Psychopharmacology

KEY POINTS

- Psychiatrists in acute care settings routinely see a significant number of patients with personality disorder pathology.
- Failure to recognize primary or co-occurring personality disorder pathology can be problematic and complicating.
- Central tenets of this evidence-based treatment (transference-focused psychotherapy [TFP]) for borderline personality disorder can be useful for clinicians in acute care settings, even when those clinicians are not acting as the primary psychotherapist.
- Utilization of fundamental principles of TFP can help improve outcomes and also serve as an effective risk management strategy.

INTRODUCTION

Transference-focused psychotherapy (TFP), one of the evidence-based treatments for patients with borderline personality disorder (BPD), was developed by clinicians steeped in psychoanalytically informed psychotherapy who recognized that their standard treatment approach required significant adjustment to be of use to patients with moderate to severe personality pathology.[1] Although TFP research has focused thus far exclusively on individual psychotherapy with those individuals meeting *Diagnostic and Statistical Manual of Mental Disorders, Fifth Edition* (DSM-5) criteria for BPD, its central principles may have utility for clinicians treating a broader group of patients and in a variety of settings including those in acute care psychiatry.[2,3] It might

---

Disclosure Statement: The author has no relationship with a commercial company that has a direct financial interest in the subject matter or materials discussed in this article.
Columbia University Medical Center, New York, NY, USA
* 25 West 81st Street, New York, NY 10024.
E-mail address: Rh170@cumc.columbia.edu

Psychiatr Clin N Am 41 (2018) 225–235
https://doi.org/10.1016/j.psc.2018.01.006
0193-953X/18/

seem, on the surface, counterintuitive to suggest using psychoanalytically informed interventions in the world of contemporary acute care psychiatry, now dominated by pharmacotherapy and cognitive-behavioral interventions. That said, numerous studies have concluded that patients with personality disorder (PD) pathology, and in particular those with BPD, are significantly represented in psychiatric emergency departments, inpatient psychiatric settings, and general outpatient psychiatric clinics.[4,5] (Although this article refers to patients with moderate to severe PD generally, because the vast majority of PD research has been on patients with BPD, most of the references relate to findings on that particular subgroup of patients.) What is the general psychiatrist's likely present-day accommodation? Some clinicians might ignore PD symptoms completely, focusing exclusively on mood, anxiety, eating, or substance use disorders, which are comorbidities frequently seen in BPD.[6] (This conjecture is supported by research examining rates of PD diagnosis in outpatient clinics; when clinicians use semistructured interviews they are much more likely to make a PD diagnosis than when assessing the same patient without such prompts.[7]) Others may try to direct patients to specialized care, although such opportunities may be rare, or prohibitively expensive, or both.[8] Applications of TFP principles, although not a panacea, can provide clinicians with a way to assess PD pathology by category and by level of severity, and to help them manage common clinical situations.

As noted, TFP was originally developed as an individual psychotherapy for patients with BPD. Since its inception, academic leaders have proposed adapting TFP concepts and techniques for patients with higher-level personality pathology, with adolescents, and with a group treatment format.[9–11] More recently, psychiatry residencies have introduced TFP teaching as a tool to enhance trainees' introduction to conducting individual psychotherapy, and as a tool to help manage patients with PD pathology in the acute care settings where residents practice.[12,13] Psychiatry residents will generally see patients in situations marked by relatively high acuity, such as emergency departments, inpatient units, and tertiary-care outpatient clinics; this acuity is associated with high rates of patients with primary PD presentations or PD symptoms co-occurring with other disorders.[14,15] In general, psychiatry residents get relatively little training about working with patients with PDs and the exposure to treatments for patients with PDs tends to be focused on dialectical behavioral therapy (DBT).[16] Although learning about DBT will certainly have utility for psychiatric trainees and assist them in considering referral options, the pilot programs introducing TFP training to residents have a broader overarching goal of integrating TFP concepts into the trainees' daily work with patients in multiple spheres.

TFP as an individual psychotherapy has a distinct way of unfolding, marked by a specific order and critical essential elements required even before the therapy begins. Once the individual psychotherapy is started, the TFP therapist will use a defined set of interventions. In this respect, TFP is unlike many "free-form" supportive or expressive psychotherapies as they are widely practiced. The notion that TFP principles can be "applied" in settings other than an extended individual psychotherapy echoes the longstanding tradition of "applied psychoanalysis" or the use of psychoanalytic theory and technique in situations outside of the individual psychotherapy dyad.[17]

THE ESSENTIAL ELEMENTS OF TRANSFERENCE-FOCUSED PSYCHOTHERAPY AS AN INDIVIDUAL PSYCHOTHERAPY

Before discussion of applications of TFP principles in acute care settings, it is useful to review the essential elements of TFP as an extended individual psychotherapy. As noted, TFP was developed by clinicians working in a psychoanalytic mode, specifically an object relations approach, who felt compelled to alter traditional psychoanalytic psychotherapy in the treatment of patients with BPD because they observed that a standard set of interventions did not seem to be effective. The overarching goal of TFP is the integration of thoughts, feelings, and actions that are "split off" or not within a patient's awareness, in the context of persistent splitting, or experiencing self and others in caricatured "all good" or "all bad" ways. The major adjustments to the traditional psychoanalytic approach included the following:

- An extended, deliberate evaluation process anchored by the structural interview, which combines assessment of both standard DSM-5 diagnostic criteria and exploration of the patient's level of organization. The short-hand term level of organization aims to capture the patient's functioning in key areas using psychodynamic terminology and understanding.[18,19]
- Discussion with the patient about the clinician's preliminary diagnostic impression, including frank discussion of PD pathology, as is the standard of care for all the evidence-based psychotherapies for BPD.[20]
- Explicit elucidation of the patient's personal goals and treatment goals. This intervention has the goal of identifying specific markers for the effectiveness of the treatment, anticipating an alternating focus on what is happening in the treatment over time and what is happening in the patient's life outside of treatment.
- A meeting held with the partner or family member in any situation in which the patient might have a significant dependence (financial, emotional) on another party. This intervention has the goal of helping the clinician (obtaining parallel information, sharing with the family member the risks associated with the disorder) and recognizing with the patient the reality of the patient's dependence, something often minimized or denied. This meeting may have the benefit of enlisting family members who become informed about and supportive of the treatment.
- An extended contracting phase, often lasting over multiple appointments, outlining the respective responsibilities of both the patient and the therapist. This process also includes exploration in advance of likely pitfalls in the treatment that may occur. The contracting phase precedes the beginning of the therapy; it is considered essential in setting the stage for the exploration of critical transference elements that are expected to emerge with the therapist, often related to the clearly outlined responsibilities.

Only when the therapist and patient have traversed the steps described, does the actual "therapy" begin. Each of these steps has multiple elements, as would be expected given the complexity of PD pathology. The following are the key guiding principles of TFP:

1. To create a situation that feels safe for both the patient *and* the therapist, and
2. To have in place a frame that will allow the patient and therapist to explore together the emerging transference currents, with close attention paid to the patient's challenges to the frame or permutations in the agreement that come from the therapist.

Once the therapy begins, the TFP clinician will follow a relatively well-defined set of interventions. These include the following:

- Monitoring the 3 channels of communication: what the patient says, how the patient behaves, and how the therapist feels.
- Tolerating the expectable confusion associated with significant PD pathology, without feeling moved to immediately organize or structure the material.

- Identifying the dominant affects that emerge in the content shared by the patient in response to the expectation that the patient speak freely about what is on his or her mind.
- Identifying the dominant object relations dyads as they emerge, or the patient's experience of self, the patient's experience of another (including the therapist), and the associated affect.
- "Naming the actors" or putting into words the therapist's initial impression of the dominant object relations dyad as it develops.
- Considering the possibility of an emerging role reversal, or evidence that the patient is behaving in a way he or she previously ascribed to others.
- Considering the way a surface dyad keeps at bay a concurrent, but less available dyad. For example, the patient experiencing himself or herself as victimized by the therapist, alternating with the patient's victimizing of the therapist, often outside of the patient's awareness. This dyad might keep at bay the patient's experience of longing for an idealized figure.
- Use of "therapist-centered interpretations" to manage episodes of patients' heightened affective reactions. Often a therapist will become defensive or argumentative in such situations. The therapist-centered interpretation invites the patient to express concern, mistrust, or even nonpsychotic paranoid thinking about the therapist.
- Repeated use of the following interventions:
  1. Clarification, or a request for more information about anything offered by the patient that is unclear or sketchy,
  2. Confrontation, or bringing to the patient's attention any conflicting or disparate data points observed in what the patient says or how the patient behaves, or
  3. Interpretation, or a preliminary hypothesis about motivations and defenses offered by the therapist to the patient for consideration.

APPLICATIONS OF TRANSFERENCE-FOCUSED PSYCHOTHERAPY PRINCIPLES IN ACUTE CARE PSYCHIATRY

The idea that TFP principles could be of use to clinicians in settings outside of an individual extended psychotherapy developed organically. Psychiatry residents learning TFP as one of a number of individual psychotherapy interventions were also fulfilling their duties in the standard tertiary-care training sites, often settings with high acuity and high rates of patients with primary or co-occurring PD pathology. These residents were thus armed with a "toolbox" of interventions to use in these settings. The "tool box" included the following:

1. Active monitoring of countertransference elements
2. Attentiveness to how the patient behaves, at least as much as to what the patient says
3. Openness to consideration of a PD diagnosis, even with incomplete information
4. Appreciation of the dominant affect expressed with words or with actions
5. Speculation about an emerging dominant object relations dyad and the possibility of role reversal

Along with these elements, TFP training gave residents some possible "scripts" to use, borrowed from TFP as an extended psychotherapy, including the following:

1. "Naming the actors"
2. Delineation of a recurrent object relations dyad and its reversal

3. The "therapist-centered interpretation" to be used in periods of heightened affect. Psychiatry trainees used these TFP principles in their work in consultation-liaison psychiatry, inpatient psychiatry treatment, and forensic psychiatry settings. Again, the goal was not to introduce a half-baked or diluted version of the individual psychotherapy, but rather to use core elements of the treatment (assessment processes, contracting, identification of patterns as reflected in dominant object relations dyads and their reversals, and maintenance of a treatment frame) in acute care settings.

It is not within the scope of this article to explore all the possible uses of TFP principles in acute care psychiatry; as noted, the literature on applied TFP thus far has introduced its use in inpatient settings (general psychiatry and forensic services), outpatient pharmacotherapy, consultation-liaison psychiatry, and crisis settings (that could include psychiatric emergency departments). This article's focus is on the use of TFP principles in prescribing for patients with primary or co-occurring moderate to severe PD pathology in a "step-down" setting, such as an intensive outpatient program. Given the shifting employment patterns among psychiatrists in the United States and Canada, and the aforementioned high rates of psychiatric comorbidity associated with serious PD diagnoses, such challenges are not rare.[21,22] What is the extent of useful training for clinicians facing such thorny challenges in contemporary practice? The situation is a murky one; there are no medications approved by the Food and Drug Administration for PD pathology. Despite this, patients with BPD, for example, are unusually high users of all subtypes of psychiatric medication.[23] Risk management education tends to be generic and does not routinely address the particular complications associated with prescribing medication to patients with PD symptoms, particularly those with subsyndromal presentations. Authoritative research groups have concluded in definitive analyses that the effectiveness of pharmacotherapy for PD symptoms is, at best, very limited.[24,25] The body governing decision-making about prescribing within the United Kingdom's National Health Service, to add to this complicated picture, has recommended use of no medications in the treatment of BPD.[26] Good Psychiatric Management for Borderline Personality Disorder (GPM), another empirically validated treatment, has specific recommendations for prescribing medications to patients with BPD, but TFP principles would extend these recommendations by (1) offering a way to think about the range of moderate to severe PD presentations, beyond those patients meeting DSM-5 criteria for BPD, and (2) providing a detailed way for the prescriber to approach treatment of the patient with PD symptoms, including attention to the level of illness severity, introduction and maintenance of a treatment frame, and introduction to a "script" when identifying and describing patterns (in TFP short-hand, the dominant object relations dyads and their reversal) and for managing episodes of heightened affective states.[27]

The following is a sample clinical vignette that aims to capture the usefulness of TFP principles for the general psychiatrist as prescriber:

Dr A is a recent psychiatry residency graduate. She takes a job with a large multi-hospital system (in current terms, an accountable care organization) that operates with a model of capitation, not fee-for-service. Her employers expect that psychiatrists in the system will prescribe medication only and refer to other professionals, mostly social workers, to provide psychotherapy in individual and group formats. Dr A is assigned to work in the intensive outpatient program, where she sees recently hospitalized patients or those outpatients seeking "crisis" appointments; she is expected to see a number of new patients per week and to see 3 patients per hour in follow-up "medication management" visits.

During her first year of practice, Dr A finds that she can manage the work load expected and she believes is able to provide quality care to her patients, with a few exceptions. Dr A notices that a relatively small number of patients in her practice, fewer than 10%, occupy a disproportionate amount of time and cause her unusual worry and uncharacteristic conflict with the other medical specialists in the hospital system and the therapists with whom she works. Dr A's residency training program had little didactic focus on PDs, just a few hours, mostly focused on DBT, taught by a psychologist. Her familiarity with the diagnosis and management of PDs, including pharmacotherapy, was limited to anecdotal information conveyed by supervisors, and the preparation she did for her psychiatry boards examination, which had few questions related to PD pathology.

Dr A learns from a friend from residency, Dr B, about the latter's experience with TFP training. Dr B has a practice that involves both psychotherapy and pharmacotherapy, and he encourages Dr A to take a 1-day TFP course, as he had done. Dr B describes his improved confidence when assessing and treating patients with complex presentations that include PD elements and reports that he uses TFP principles in multiple clinical situations other than an extended individual psychotherapy.

Dr A takes the TFP course and begins to integrate into her work elements of the treatment she has learned.

POINT 1: ASSESSMENT

The TFP assessment process is based on the structural interview. This process, first described decades ago, presaged the current hybrid categorical-dimensional approach of the DSM-5 appendix.[28] The structural interview aims to capture not just the diagnostic category (borderline PD, narcissistic PD), but also how impaired or functional the patient is. The structural interview has the goal of investigating the following elements, easily remembered using the mnemonic RADIOS:

- Reality testing
- Aggression
- Defenses (specifically the admixture of mature, repression-based, or splitting based defenses)
- Identity diffusion versus consolidation
- Object relations (the nature and quality of the patient's connections with others)
- Superego functioning (or moral values)

The TFP assessment process also attempts to identify elements that might suggest a particularly concerning prognosis, specifically a "secondary gain" of the patient's illness, or some elements of prominent aggression, nonpsychotic paranoia, or antisocial traits. The term secondary gain of illness captures those patients whose symptoms and condition confer some kind of gratification, which can be in the patient's awareness, or sometimes not. Such situations could include the exploitative patient who gets financial support from family or the state based on his or her psychiatric symptoms. Another example would be the patient who derives gratification from the sympathy derived from or control over family members who "walk on eggshells" because of the patient's condition. The patient with elements of ego-syntonic aggression, nonpsychotic paranoia, and antisocial traits may have a subtype of severe narcissistic PD pathology that would alert the clinician about likely challenges going forward with the treatment.

Dr A begins to incorporate certain TFP assessment elements in her initial evaluation of patients. She moves from a "decision-tree" approach to one informed by the structural interview. She spends more time on elements of the patient's social history, at times, and pays particular attention to issues of finances and legal difficulties, when indicated. Dr A begins to use the RADIOS mnemonic in her thinking, aiming to gage how functional or impaired each patient might be, often using her countertransference to consider a patient's aggression or aspects of the patient's defensive operations as they emerge in their budding relationship.

POINT 2: SHARING THE PERSONALITY DISORDER DIAGNOSIS

Dr A had learned during her residency that it was not appropriate to make a PD diagnosis when other co-occurring disorders were active. During her first year in practice, this policy seemed to Dr A impractical; a number of her most challenging patients had both PD symptoms and co-occurring mood, anxiety, substance use, or eating disorders that often showed no signs of remitting any time soon. Dr A learned in her TFP training that ignoring PD symptoms and/or withholding PD diagnoses from patients and families might not be in anyone's best interest.

Dr A slowly began to introduce to certain patients her understanding of the contribution of PD symptoms or diagnoses to their difficulties. In some cases, she used standard DSM-5 terminology; in other cases, Dr A used more euphemistic language, as when describing to a patient with a "thin-skinned" narcissistic disorder profile the likelihood that his mood reactivity might be best understood as related to fluctuations in his self-esteem. Making a PD diagnosis and then sharing her impressions with patients and families allowed Dr A to qualify her endorsement of certain medication trials and even recommend stopping certain medications. Dr A also found making and sharing PD disorder diagnoses allowed her to engage in a more honest informed consent process and limited the situations in which patients were disappointed with the results of medication trials, a familiar pattern she had noticed during her first year of practice.

POINT 3: FAMILY INVOLVEMENT

The standard TFP approach to beginning an individual psychotherapy will strongly encourage a family meeting in situations in which patients are dependent on partners or parents in some significant way. Given TFP's development as a treatment for BPD, these situations were not rare; such patients often function poorly and require significant emotional or financial support, or have destructive enmeshed relationships, often a source of confusion for the treaters involved. In addition, because many patients with BPD are actively suicidal, treaters often experience understandable anxiety about these patients, made worse when treaters feel isolated or "in the dark" because patients forbid contact with family members. The family meeting in TFP has multiple goals: to help the therapist as he or she gathers parallel information; to address risk management elements, as family members are given an opportunity to raise their concerns; and to address an often-unspoken aspect of the patient's denial, that his or her disorder has led to a state of dependence.

Dr A begins a treatment with Mr C who presents in a "crisis appointment." He comes with a diagnosis of "treatment-resistant depression" and has failed numerous medication trials and psychotherapies. Mr C comes to Dr A on an unusually complex regimen that includes a monoamine oxidase inhibitor (MAOI) antidepressant and a relatively high benzodiazepine dose. Mr C has not worked for a number of years; he recently moved back in with his parents who are paying toward his health insurance. Dr A's initial assessment suggested Mr C had significant PD pathology in the narcissistic category, along with his purported depressive disorder. Dr A was aware of her own countertransference, both irritated by Mr C's entitlement and fearful about his adherence to the MAOI diet, given his history of 2 recent emergency room visits following his impulsive decision to try eating pizza.

Dr A feels strongly she would need to have a meeting with Mr C and his family if she were to feel comfortable enough to continue their treatment. Mr C was somewhat reluctant to have the meeting, but eventually agreed. During the meeting, Dr A was able to learn more about Mr C, which confirmed her initial impression about co-occurring narcissistic PD traits, and she was able to explain to Mr C's parents her goals for the treatment and the risks associated with his current regimen. Following the meeting, Dr C felt more comfortable going forward treating Mr C, as she had clearly reviewed the risks associated with his underlying disorder and the medications he had been prescribed begun by prior clinicians.

POINT 4: NEGOTIATING THE TREATMENT CONTRACT

The TFP contract anchors the extended psychotherapy; this contract is more than "boiler plate" office policies, it outlines the patient's and the therapist's responsibilities and initiates a discussion of likely challenges to the treatment frame, as would be expected with patients with moderate to severe PD symptoms. The contract should include all the details necessary so that the clinician can feel secure in his or her treatment; the goal is for the clinician to be able to think clearly and not feel clouded by undue anxiety. The contracting phase follows the evaluation process; the general rule of thumb is that the more impaired the patient is (in TFP parlance, the lower the level of organization), the more rigorous the treatment frame. Many clinicians, including prescribers, will take a one-size-fits-all approach. Unfortunately, what might work when prescribing medication for a patient with a generally higher level of organization (operating without a treatment contract) can lead to confusion, surprise, or even outright panic for the psychiatrist or nurse practitioner responsible for treating patients with more significant PD pathology. The act of establishing a treatment contract will proactively address a well-described phenomenon among patients with PD: a belief, conscious or unconscious, that a prescriber and the medications he or she recommends will be enough on their own to address a chronic PD condition. A patient may express surprise that he or she has *any* responsibility in his or her treatment; a detailed treatment contract will introduce this reality from the beginning.

The following is a list of TFP contracting elements that will have salience for the prescriber who may *not* be engaged in psychotherapy:

- Scheduling process
- Starting and stopping sessions on time
- Patient hygiene
- Fee and payment schedule
- Cancellation policy
- Intersession contact
- Permission to contact family members
- Permission to contact other treaters
- Adherence with medical care
- Adherence with laboratory testing
- Adherence with medication
- A requirement for abstinence from substance abuse, if indicated
- A plan for managing eating disorder symptoms, if indicated
- Participation in adjunctive treatments
- The patient's obligation to be honest

- Management of suicidal behavior
- Involvement of psychiatric emergency services
- Involvement of psychiatric inpatient services

Ms D is discharged from the inpatient psychiatric unit to Dr A's care. Ms D was hospitalized briefly following an episode that was initially understood as a suicide gesture; she had taken 4 times the recommended dose of her sleeping medication, apparently in the context of an argument with her boyfriend. (She later denied any intent to harm herself.) Dr A notes that the chart from the inpatient hospitalization lists diagnoses including primary insomnia, unspecified anxiety disorder, and unspecified PD. Dr A also reads about Ms D's most recent treatment, which was marked by nonadherence to her medication regimen, missed appointments, and premature calls for medication refills.

Dr A's initial evaluation of Ms D suggested some prominent BPD symptoms associated with the hospitalization, specifically affective instability, unstable interpersonal relationships, and a preoccupation with abandonment. Dr A was aware of her immediate countertransference, feeling anxiety (Would Ms D misuse her medications again?) and irritation (Would she be subject to complaints from Ms D if she did not comply with premature requests for refills? Would Ms D lodge a complaint with the accountable care organization, something taken seriously by administrators?) Dr A felt strongly that her best hope for treating Ms D would rest on a wide-ranging and detailed contract. Dr A spent a significant portion of her initial sessions with Ms D putting this contract together. She expected push-back from Ms D, which she got, but remained clear that an agreement in place would be necessary. As the treatment progressed, Dr A referred back to the contract repeatedly, and monitored her own urges to depart from the contract as they came up.

POINT 5: IDENTIFYING DOMINANT OBJECT RELATIONS DYADS AND THEIR REVERSAL

TFP as a psychotherapy provides clinicians with certain explicit "scripts" that are used to explore recurrent object relations dyads as they emerge in the course of treatment. The TFP therapist first attempts to "name the actors" or put into words the most prominent object relations dyad in evidence, often a challenge when obscured by the chaos so often prominent with a severe PD disorder. The therapist then continues to refine this object relations dyad, often highlighting the patient's experience of the therapist, while observing for a role reversal, or the way the patient might behave in a way he or she previously ascribed to others. Sometime in periods of heightened affective states, or "affect storms," the therapist will simply put into words the particular stark experience of the therapist the patient is having at the time. The affect storm is often marked by the patient's mistrustful or devaluing sentiments about the therapist. These "scripts" may be of use to the prescriber in ongoing treatment, given the likelihood that medications will have powerful and complicated meaning for the patient with PD.

Dr A meets weekly with Ms D in the period following her hospitalization. Ms D continues to have difficulty sleeping, despite Dr A's review of sleep hygiene guidelines and a referral for cognitive-behavioral therapy specific for insomnia. Ms D presents to her next appointment looking angry, sitting with her arms crossed and scowling. She is sarcastic with Dr A, stating "Those new pills you gave me for sleep are pretty worthless. You took away the narcotic–the one thing that helped me sleep. I didn't sleep a wink last night and now I have to go to work feeling terrible!" Dr A attempts to "name the actors" in this exchange, guessing at what Ms D is going through. She responds: "It sounds like you're feeling pretty vulnerable, seeing me as not very competent or maybe just uncaring, and you're pretty upset about it." This comment was momentarily containing. Later in their meeting, Ms D is more aggressive, raising her voice and threatening Dr A that if she can't get a good night sleep, she may need to take an excessive dose of medication as she had before, risking rehospitalization. Dr A avoids an excessively active response to this comment, instead describing the dominant object relations she observes, and its reversal, by saying: "You've made it clear you see yourself as neglected and powerless, suspecting that I'm acting in a punishing way; I'm also aware that right now your threats about adherence to your medication regimen and a risk of rehospitalization are punishing to me, likely to concern me or even frighten me." Dr A considered that putting her observation into words did not immediately lead Ms D to have an increased insight into her behavior, but it did diffuse the threat in the air, thereby reducing Dr A's anxiety.

SUMMARY

TFP principles applied outside of an individual psychotherapy modality have a practical utility for psychiatrists working in acute care settings. Psychiatric education about work with patients with PD diagnoses is limited, at best. Psychiatrists will work with patients with PD diagnoses in almost all the settings where they practice, and such work is bound to be fraught and labor-intensive. TFP principles offer a commonsensical and organizing blueprint for psychiatrists. Its systematic approach, deliberate and considered, can help psychiatrists in practice manage some of their most challenging clinical situations.

REFERENCES

1. Yeomans F, Clarkin J, Kernberg O. Transference-focused psychotherapy for borderline personality disorder: a clinical guide. Washington, DC: American Psychiatric Publishing; 2015.
2. Hersh R, Caligor E, Yeomans F. Fundamentals of transference-focused psychotherapy: applications in psychiatric and medical settings. Cham (Switzerland): Springer; 2017.
3. Hersh R. Using transference-focused psychotherapy principles in the pharmacotherapy of patients with severe personality disorders. Psychodyn Psychiatry 2015;43(2):181–200.
4. Zimmerman MD, Chelminski I, Young D. The frequency of personality disorder in psychiatric patients. Psychiatr Clin 2008;31(3):405–20.
5. Hong V. Borderline personality disorder in the emergency department: good psychiatric management. Harv Rev Psychiatry 2016;24(5):357–66.
6. Paris J. Why psychiatrists are reluctant to diagnose: borderline personality disorder. Psychiatry 2007;4(1):35–9.
7. Zimmerman M, Mattia J. Differences between clinical and research practices in diagnosing borderline personality disorder. Am J Psychiatry 1999;156(10):1570–4.
8. Paris J. Stepped care and rehabilitation for patients recovering from borderline personality disorder. J Clin Psychol 2015;71(8):747–52.
9. Caligor E, Kernberg O, Clarkin J. Handbook of dynamic psychotherapy for higher level personality pathology. Washington, DC: American Psychiatric Publishing; 2007.
10. Normandin L, Ensink K. Transference-focused psychotherapy for borderline adolescents: a neurobiologically informed psychotherapy. J Infant Child Adolesc Psychother 2015;14(1):98–110.

11. Kernberg O. The inseparable nature of love and aggression: clinical and theoretical perspectives. Arlington (VA): American Psychiatric Publishing; 2012.
12. Bernstein J, Zimmerman M, Auchincloss E. Transference-focused psychotherapy training during residency: an aide to learning psychodynamic psychotherapy. Psychodyn Psychiatry 2015;43(2):201–22.
13. Zerbo E, Cohen S, Bielska W, et al. Transference-focused psychotherapy in the general psychiatry residency: a useful and applicable model for residents in acute care settings. Psychodyn Psychiatry 2013;41(1):163–81.
14. Pascual J, Corcoles D, Castano J, et al. Hospitalization and pharmacotherapy for borderline personality disorder in a psychiatric emergency service. Psychiatr Serv 2007;58:1199–204.
15. Bender D, Dolan R, Skodol A, et al. Treatment utilization by patients with personality disorders. Am J Psychiatry 2001;158(2):295–302.
16. Sansone R, Kay J, Anderson J. Resident education in borderline personality disorder: is it sufficient? Acad Psychiatry 2013;37(4):287–8.
17. Gourgechon P. Typology of applied psychoanalysis. Int J Appl Psychoanal Stud 2013;10(3):192–8.
18. Kernberg OF. Structural interviewing. Psychiatr Clin 1981;4:169–95.
19. Kernberg OF. Severe personality disorders: psychotherapeutic strategies. New Haven (CT): Yale University Press; 1984.
20. Weinberg I, Ronningstam E, Goldblatt MJ, et al. Common factors in empirically supported treatments of borderline personality disorder. Curr Psychiatry Rep 2011;13(1):60–8.
21. Fiester S, Ellison JM, Docherty JP, et al. Comorbidity of personality disorders: two for the price of one. New Dir Ment Health Serv 1990;47:103–14.
22. Mojtabai R, Olfson M. National trends in psychotherapy by office-based psychiatrists. Arch Gen Psychiatry 2008;65(8):962–70.
23. Zanarini M, Frankenburg F, Hennen J, et al. Mental health service utilization by borderline personality disorder patients and axis II comparison subjects followed prospectively for 6 years. J Clin Psychol 2004;65(1):28–36.
24. Khalifa N, Duggan C, Stoffers, et al. Pharmacological interventions for antisocial personality disorder. Cochrane Database Syst Rev 2014;(8):CD007667.
25. Stoffers J, Vollm BA, Rucker G, et al. Pharmacologic interventions for borderline personality disorder. Cochrane Database Syst Rev 2010;(6):CD005653.
26. National Institute for Health and Clinical Excellence (NICE). Borderline personality disorder, treatment and management. London: The British Psychologist Society and the Royal College of Psychiatrists; 2009. Available at: www.nice.org.uk/cg78.
27. Gunderson J, Links P. Handbook of good psychiatric management for borderline personality disorder. Washington, DC: American Psychiatric Publishing; 2014.
28. Oldham JM. The alternative DSM-5 model for personality disorder. World Psychiatry 2015;14(2):234–6.

Psychodynamic Psychiatry, the Biopsychosocial Model, and the Difficult Patient

Eric M. Plakun, MD

KEYWORDS

- Difficult patient • Biopsychosocial model • Enactment
- Treatment-resistant disorders • Psychodynamic psychiatry

KEY POINTS

- Psychodynamic psychiatry is the intersection between general psychiatry and psychoanalysis as a theory of mind, and is built on a biopsychosocial model for understanding and treating mental disorders.
- The biomedical model has not lived up to its promise and is not supported by emerging science as robustly as is the biopsychosocial model.
- The "difficult patient" emerges in part from the limits of our treatment models and treatment methods.

INTRODUCTION

Psychiatry is the medical specialty that focuses on disorders of the mind, especially disturbances in thinking, behavior, and emotions. Psychoanalysis refers here not to a form of individual psychotherapy, but rather to a theory of mind that attends to an individual's unique developmental trajectory within a familial and cultural context, with attention to the important impact of unconscious factors on human thought and behavior. Given these 2 definitions, we can think of psychodynamic psychiatry as the area of intersection between the domain of psychoanalysis as a theory of mind and the domain of general psychiatry. Psychodynamic psychiatry offers a perspective that allows us to engage, understand, and be useful to difficult-to-treat patients.[1]

All of us have experienced work with patients we come to view as difficult to treat or, as they are sometimes called, "treatment resistant."[2] There are patient-specific and disorder-specific characteristics that make patients difficult to treat, but that which is difficult often resides not in them, but in us, and in the limitations of our treatments.

No disclosures.

Austen Riggs Center, 25 Main Street, Stockbridge, MA 01262, USA
E-mail address: Eric.Plakun@austenriggs.net

Psychiatr Clin N Am 41 (2018) 237–248
https://doi.org/10.1016/j.psc.2018.01.007

Abbreviations	
BPD	Borderline personality disorder
CBT	Cognitive behavioral therapy
DSM	Diagnostic and Statistical Manual of Mental Disorders
PDT	Psychodynamic therapy
RCT	Randomized controlled trials
RDoC	Research domain criteria
STAR*D	Sequenced Treatment Alternatives to Relieve Depression

This article is in 2 sections that each address different kinds of limitations that contribute to the experience of patients as difficult. The first section addresses limits inherent in the biomedical model that threatens to supplant the biopsychosocial model, which is better supported by research and more salient for understanding and treating mental disorders. The second section elaborates the way our inevitable human vulnerability to countertransference enactments contributes to the experience of patients as difficult.

LIMITATIONS OF THE BIOMEDICAL MODEL

Mathematician George Box noted that, "All models are wrong, but some are useful."[3] It was George Engel[4] who proposed the biopsychosocial model, a model suggesting that understanding and treating people with mental disorders requires attention to the contributions of their biology, individual psychology, and social context. The biopsychosocial model is entirely congruent with psychodynamic psychiatry. However, over the last several decades, a narrower biomedical model has been in ascendancy and the biopsychosocial model has been in decline. Popular psychiatrist authors like Nasir Ghaemi, for example, have criticized the biopsychosocial model as lacking rigor.[5]

There was hope in the 1990s that the eventual decoding of the human genome and findings from brain research would confirm the value of a biomedical model. Current director of the National Institutes of Health, Francis Collins, who was then director of the National Human Genome Research Institute, suggested in 1999 that a genetic revolution throughout medicine would emerge from the Human Genome Project. At that time, Collins[6] described 6 major outcomes expected to follow from decoding the human genome:

1. Common diseases will be explained largely by a few DNA variants with strong associations to disease;
2. This knowledge will lead to improved diagnosis;
3. Such knowledge will also drive preventive medicine;
4. Pharmacogenomics will improve therapeutic decision making;
5. Gene therapy will treat multiple diseases; and
6. A substantial increase in novel targets for drug development and therapy will ensue.

Although there are some small advances toward achieving these outcomes in the rest of medicine, in psychiatry the promise has fallen short. Associated with these hopes for the future are 3 implicit assumptions related to the biomedical model:

1. Genes equal disease,
2. Patients present with single disorders that respond to specific evidence based treatments, and
3. The best treatments are pills.

As it turns out, however, these assumptions are not supported by the emerging data. As Box[3] suggests, both models are inevitably wrong, but emerging research more strongly supports the biopsychosocial model than the biomedical model.

In neuroscience, research has tended to associate multiple disorders with the same brain regions—usually the prefrontal cortex, amygdala, anterior cingulate cortex, and some others. In the absence of clear evidence that psychopathology is localized to specific brain regions, interest has shifted toward understanding how the "connectome" functions in states of mental health and disease.

Genes Equal Disease

Despite Collins' predictions, we have not found genes that cause most common mental disorders. In genome-wide association study studies of depression, using samples large enough to discover relevant single nucleotide polymorphisms involved in some medical disorders, 17 single nucleotide polymorphisms account for only a small amount of the variance in heritability of depression,[7] whereas in schizophrenia more than 125 single nucleotide polymorphisms have been detected, and some of these are found across disorders.[8] The most significant schizophrenia single nucleotide polymorphism is a C4 gene variant related to synaptic pruning, which is associated with an increase in the base rate of schizophrenia from 1% to 1.25%.[9] Copy number variation studies show that spontaneous mutations account for roughly 2% of the variance in causation of schizophrenia.[10]

Although mental disorders are clearly heritable, other research reveals the importance of psychosocial factors. The presence of major depressive disorder in mothers during childrearing increases the risk of depression in their adolescent biological and adopted children.[11] Similarly, in twin mothers with anxiety disorders, the transmission of anxiety to their offspring was better accounted for by environmental than genetic factors.[12]

Although no genetic or other biomarkers have been found for mental disorders, early adverse experiences have emerged as an "enviromarker" associated with an increased risk of 1 or more mental or substance use disorders, and with more medical disorders.[13,14]

There is widespread acknowledgment that the genetics of mental disorders are complex and polygenic, and that there is not a simple equation of genes equal disease. Some have begun to question the underlying biomedical brain and genomics focused "big idea" that drives theory and research funding.[15] The field has shifted toward study of "gene-by-environment interactions," which is just another way of saying "biopsychosocial."

Patients Present with Single Disorders That Respond to Specific Evidence-Based Treatment

Although practice guidelines from the American Psychiatric Association are written for 1 disorder at a time, we have learned that the presence of multiple comorbid disorders is the rule rather than the exception in clinical populations. For example, Wisniewski and colleagues[16] found that 78% of patients from the large, multisite Sequenced Treatment Alternatives to Relieve Depression (STAR*D) study of depression had comorbidity or suicidal ideation that would exclude them from randomized controlled trials (RCTs) of treatment for depression. Although we test treatments for depression on specially selected groups of patients, such patients are not representative of the majority who present in clinical settings. In the STAR*D sample, the larger group of depressed patients generally excluded from RCTs was less tolerant of medication, and had lower rates of treatment response (39% vs 52%) and remission (25% vs

34%). Comorbid depressed patients represent 1 segment of the group of difficult patients—difficult because they do not respond as well to evidence-based treatments as we might expect from RCTs testing treatments on noncomorbid patients.

Another group of difficult patients is those with borderline personality disorder (BPD) and other personality disorders. Although part of what makes patients with BPD difficult to treat is the immature defenses that engage us in enactments, as described elsewhere in this article, our relative blindness to the presence or impact of BPD also plays a role, because we cannot treat what we will not see.

In the Collaborative Longitudinal Personality Disorder study, the presence of a personality disorder adversely affected depression outcome, caused persistent functional impairment, and extensive treatment use, and was associated with significant suicide risk.[17,18] The presence of personality disorders, especially BPD, "robustly predicted persistence" of major depression.[19] Skodol and colleagues[17] thus call for careful assessment of the presence of personality disorders in depressed patients. However, the most frequent personality disorder diagnosis offered in the *Diagnostic and Statistical Manual of Mental Disorders* (DSM)-IV was "deferred," a common practice of clinicians that leaves them blind to what may be making a patient difficult to treat—and leaves such depressed patients with undiagnosed comorbid BPD without effective treatment.

- "Difficult" patients may have undiagnosed comorbid BPD.
- We cannot treat what we will not see.

The reality that patients tend to have multiple comorbid disorders and that comorbidity predicts a greater likelihood of "treatment resistance" suggests that there are limits to our current diagnostic system as codified, even in the most recent versions of the DSM and *International Classification of Disease*. This recognition led Tom Insel, former director of the National Institutes of Mental Health, to launch the research domain criteria (RDoC) matrix in an effort to think beyond traditional diagnostic categories that overlap and lack specificity. The RDoC matrix includes behavior, emotion, cognition, motivation, social behavior, genes, molecules, and neural circuits. A move beyond the DSM categories makes sense, given the absence of clear links between brain mechanisms or genetic findings and clinically familiar diagnostic categories; but RDoC searches for biomarkers—a search some have likened to that for the Holy Grail—with little opportunity provided in the RDoC matrix for the role of environmental factors like relationships and attachment within gene-by-environment interactions.

Recognizing that most patients have multiple comorbid disorders, that the same brain circuitry is implicated across disorders, and that we use the same drugs for multiple disorders, Caspi and colleagues[20] tested their hypothesis that 3 underlying factors (externalizing, internalizing, and thought disorders) account for all mental disorders in a sample of more than 1000 patients whose symptoms were followed for 20 years. Although there was some statistical support for the 3-factor model of mental disorders, a better fit was found for a 1-factor model. Calling this factor "p" for psychopathology, Caspi and colleagues note that those with a high p are at significantly greater risk for 1 or more mental or substance use disorders over time, with the opposite true for those with low p. Further, p seemed to be a function of compromised early brain development, early and recent adversity, and a family history of a mental disorder.

The findings from Caspi and associates suggest that diagnostic categories as we know them are a surface representation. An analogy to mountain ranges helps to clarify this. Those who know the Alps know Mont Blanc or the Matterhorn by their distinctive silhouettes, just as we know major depression or schizophrenia by their distinctive surface representation. However, in the case of both mountains and diagnostic categories, they are really the result of unseen forces, whether these forces are collisions between tectonic plates and erosion owing to wind and water or, in the case of diagnoses, p. Diagnostic categories as we know them seem to be surface illusions built by unseen forces.

> The research Caspi and coworkers have conducted suggests diagnostic categories as we know them are surface illusions built by unseen forces.

The Best Treatments Are Pills

Consistent with the biomedical model, much of psychiatric practice has shifted toward diagnosis and prescribing in 15-minute medication checks—with some of that time spent interfacing with an electronic health record rather than the patient. Prescribing medications is seen by some as the best we have to offer, but data from RCTs reveals their significant limitations. Caspi and colleagues accurately observed that we tend to use the same medications for all disorders. And, as noted, in the STAR*D study, RCT exclusion criteria mean that antidepressant drugs work for a minority of those seeking treatment. Meanwhile, the efficacy of antidepressants has been overestimated by about one-third when unpublished studies are included in analyses,[21] and the placebo effect accounts for as much as 75% of their benefit.[22] In the case of psychotic disorders, the Clinical Antipsychotic Trials of Intervention Effectiveness (CATIE) study shows us that patients do not find the benefit of our medications worth the risks.[23] In bipolar disorder, the Systematic Treatment Enhancement Program for Bipolar Disorder (STEP-BD) study suggests more is going on in this disorder than can be corrected by prescription of mood-stabilizing and neuroleptic medications.[24] Although the biomedical model teaches us to regard medications as psychiatry's primary treatment modality, such tunnel vision contributes to biologically focused treatment strategies that are inadequate and thus contribute to patients becoming difficult or treatment resistant. Simply put, often the source of a patient's treatment resistance lies in us.

> - Although the biomedical model teaches us to regard medications as psychiatry's primary treatment modality, such tunnel vision contributes to biologically focused treatment strategies that are inadequate and contribute to patients becoming difficult or treatment resistant.
> - Often the source of a patient's treatment resistance lies in us.

The use of a biopsychosocial rather than a biomedical model invites us to include other ways of understanding and treating psychopathology beyond biology. More than 1000 studies demonstrate the efficacy of cognitive behavioral therapy (CBT) and 200 the efficacy of psychodynamic therapy (PDT) for a range of individual and complex comorbid disorders. CBT researchers have often taken the lead in providing research evidence, but a recent high-quality metaanalysis shows the equivalence of

PDT to CBT for a range of disorders—using therapists with allegiance to the therapies tested and without sham therapy comparisons that are intended to fail,[25] as when Gilboa-Schechtman and coworkers[26] compared prolonged exposure for posttraumatic stress disorder with sham PDT that required PDT therapists to change the subject if patients discussed their trauma.

Consistent with the limitations of diagnosis and the reality of comorbidity, Barlow and colleagues[27] recently published a study of so-called unified protocol CBT, which targets not the symptoms of specific disorders, but underlying emotional dysregulation and neuroticism, demonstrating this form of CBT was as effective as disorder specific CBT for anxiety disorders. Psychoanalysis was the first unified protocol treatment to target underlying psychopathology rather than the surface disorder, but, as is so often the case, it is CBT therapists who took the lead in designing and conducting studies.

In summary, the biomedical model limits us as clinicians because genes do not equal disease, most patients have multiple comorbid disorders, there are high failure rates even for our evidence-based treatments, and BPD is underdiagnosed and thus undertreated. The biomedical model leads us to pursue biology when emerging science suggests we should be mindful of complexity, gene-by-environment interactions and a biopsychosocial perspective. These shortcomings of the biomedical model contribute to the proportion of patients perceived as difficult.

- The biomedical model limits us as clinicians because genes do not equal disease, most patients have multiple comorbid disorders, there are high failure rates even for our evidence-based treatments, and BPD is underdiagnosed and undertreated.
- The biomedical model leads us to pursue biology when emerging science suggests we should be mindful of complexity, gene-by-environment interactions and a biopsychosocial perspective.

ENACTMENT: A CO-CREATED PSYCHOSOCIAL MECHANISM THAT MAKES PATIENTS DIFFICULT

One reason patients are experienced as difficult is their engagement of us in ways that leave us feeling confused, hurt, angry, guilty, lost, or all of these. We might wonder, "What's going on here? Why does this patient have to be so 'difficult'?" It is the propensity to evoke such feelings in treaters that makes patients with BPD, for example, so stigmatized—disliked, avoided, and seen as difficult—with the term borderline sometimes hurled as an epithet. Patients with BPD and other personality disorders have a unique ability to get under our skin in unpleasant ways that contribute to our experience of them as difficult. When this happens, we and they are often caught up in a process called an enactment by psychodynamic psychiatrists. Enactment is formally defined as "a pattern of non-verbal interactional behavior between 2 parties in a therapeutic situation."[28] Understanding enactments offers an opportunity to untangle difficult interactions and be of more use to patients, with more equanimity in ourselves.

The origin of such experiences with patients is in their immature defenses—and the way they engage our own. Humans, including those with BPD, and those who treat patients, deploy a range of defenses from the more mature (eg, intellectualization, sublimation, humor) to the more immature (eg, splitting, projective identification, acting out). Those with BPD differ from most of us who do treatment by virtue of the greater frequency with which they deploy immature defenses like projective identification, which is the relevant defense to understanding enactment.

From Projective Identification to Enactment

The simplest definition of projective identification involves patients putting into us (ie, projecting) a disavowed affect that represents elements of their life history. In this definition, our role is passive—like an antenna picking up a transmitted signal. The following case example illustrates this definition.

Case Vignette for Projective Identification

A 30-year-old man in weekly PDT for feelings of self-doubt receives a reduced fee from his woman therapist. In the course of therapy, he meets and decides to marry a wealthy woman, but struggles in therapy with worry that he is marrying her for money rather than love. When the woman therapist raises the reduced fee after the marriage, as she said she would, the patient is enraged at the therapist's greediness.

In this example of projective identification, the patient struggling with self-doubt disavows fear of his own potential greediness and finds it in the therapist.

Of course, simple definitions are just that, and in reality projective identification is more complex. That is, the other onto whom the projection is placed has some kind of "hook" on which the projection can be hung. We unwittingly accept the projection because of this hook that comes from our own character and life history. In the case vignette, this hook might be the therapist's discomfort with being seen as greedy, especially when she raises the fee.

However, things get even more complicated when we remember that projective identification is an immature defense used by all humans to differing degrees. And therapists are decidedly human. When both parties in a therapeutic situation are involved in mutual and complementary projective identification—a patient disavowing an unacceptable affect and putting it on a hook in the therapist, and a therapist reciprocally disavowing an unacceptable affect and putting it on a hook in the patient—then they are in an enactment.[29]

An "enactment" is a set of mutual and complementary projective identifications involving both participants in a therapeutic situation, and informed by the life histories of both participants.

We can see the transition from projective identification to enactment by returning to the case vignette and adding a bit more detail.

Case Vignette for Enactment

A 30-year-old man in weekly PDT for feelings of self-doubt receives a reduced fee from his woman therapist. Both are therapists, but the patient works in a low-fee community mental health setting for a low salary, whereas the therapist is in a lucrative private practice—and struggles throughout the treatment with countertransference guilt about the difference between their levels of compensation for similar work. In the course of therapy, the patient meets and decides to marry a wealthy woman, but struggles in therapy with worry that he is marrying her for money rather than love. When the woman therapist raises the reduced fee after the marriage, as she said she would, the patient is enraged at the therapist's greediness. The therapist feels she is doing the sensible thing, but also feels guilty, and repeatedly makes accounting mistakes in preparing bills for the patient—sometimes overcharging and sometimes undercharging.

We can see how each party in the enactment is caught projecting something disavowed, while finding a hook in the other to hang it on. The result is a tangled engagement that is difficult for both. Sometimes enactments like these lead to fights or impasses in therapy, but they also offer an opportunity to grasp something important in the entanglement and deepen understanding and engagement between the parties.

Enactments are ubiquitous and inevitable therapeutic phenomena. They are not limited to dynamic psychotherapy, but occur in prescribing relationships, on treatment teams, and in hospital or clinic systems. In individual work with patients, whether therapy or other clinical work, enactments are most common when immature defenses are most common, as in work with patients with BPD or those with early adverse experiences involving previous caretakers that affects new caretaker relationships. Enactments may be isolated events, but in work with enactment-prone patients, enactments are often the terrain over which treatment progresses. Our task is not simply to avoid them, but to learn to use them.

Skiing offers a useful analogy for enactments in therapeutic situations. In both skiing and therapy, one is on a slippery slope. As in skiing, sliding down hill on the slippery slope is expected—even inevitable. What separates experienced from inexperienced skiers, and therapists, is how well they find their edges as they slide down hill, so that they can control the speed of their slide to stay in control and avoid crashing.[30] Finding ones edges, that is, learning to use enactments, is addressed elsewhere in this article.

Patients with Abuse Histories as Difficult Patients

Psychodynamic therapists and psychodynamic psychiatrists learn to operate from a stance of nonjudgmental, warm, and empathic technical neutrality. Technical neutrality does not imply that the therapist or other clinician is distant, uncaring, silent, or uninvolved. Psychodynamic clinicians learn to "take" the transference that is offered, that is, they tolerate the transference the patient brings into the work and the associated countertransference. However, some transferences are hard to take, and therapists and other clinicians often enter enactments by unwittingly refusing or actualizing the transference. This is a special problem with the group of difficult patients with histories of abuse.

In work with patients with abuse histories there are 3 readily available transference roles for the therapist or other clinician: perpetrator of abuse, victim of abuse, and silent witness who tolerates abuse.[31] Refusal or actualization of these transferences leads to predictable patterns of enactment illustrated in **Table 1**.

When the transference is to the clinician as perpetrator of abuse, actualizing the transference may lead the clinician unwittingly to become abusive, sadistic, and unempathic. If the perpetrator transference is refused, that is, if the clinician has trouble tolerating being seen as a perpetrator of abuse, he or she may become excessively kind and solicitous, demonstrating how much he or she cares for the patient, sometimes in extreme cases leading to "loving" boundary violations, including extending sessions and even sexual boundary violations.

When the transference is to the clinician as victim of abuse, actualizing the transference may be associated with masochistic and guilty surrender to mistreatment by an abusive patient, which may contribute to burnout from "vicarious traumatization" in work with such patients. If the clinician as victim transference is refused, we may see the clinician counterattack or abruptly terminate in a refusal to allow such work to continue.

When the transference is to the clinician as silent witness who tolerates or ignores abuse, actualizing the transference may lead to the clinician becoming

Table 1
Refusing and actualizing transferences with patients who have experienced abuse

Transference to Therapist in Role of →	Perpetrator	Victim	Silent Witness
Result if transference is actualized	• Therapist becomes abusive • In extreme cases, "sadistic" boundary violations • Overmedicates	• Therapist in masochistic surrender • Guilty • Burnout from "vicarious traumatization"	• Therapist distant • Unempathic • Uninvolved • Dissociated • Overmedicates
Result if transference is refused	• Therapist becomes excessively kind, solicitous • In extreme cases, "loving" boundary violations • Overmedicates	• Counterattacks • Termination • Overmedicates	• Overzealous rescuer, may overmedicate • Intolerance of not knowing, with im planting of false memories

distant, unempathic, uninvolved, and dissociated in the work. If the silent witness transference is refused, we may see the clinician become an overzealous rescuer, and intolerance of not knowing may lead to implanting of false memories of abuse that create pseudocertainty about that which cannot really be known.

For psychiatrists caught in refusing or actualizing these transferences with difficult patients, overmedication of the patient is a frequent result, as if to medicate away the transference such difficult patients bring into the encounter.

Using Enactments

The capacity to use enactments involves 3 steps: detect, analyze, and use the enactment.[30] We detect enactments by attending to our free-floating responsiveness in sessions. Analysis of enactments requires unpacking their meaning. What are we caught in? What are the bits of projective identification unfolding between therapist and patient? Analyzing an enactment requires that one know one's blind spots and hooks, and often is facilitated by consultation with a colleague or supervision. Using an enactment may involve engaging a patient in serious discussion of the details of what you are both caught in, with due caution about undue disclosure of the therapist's life history. Often the unpacking of an enactment, with each party owning their role in the tangled situation that has emerged, leads to a deeper and more intimate engagement. In other situations, therapists may simply realize they are caught in repeating behavior that they need to understand, contain, and stop repeating, without necessarily discussing the issue with the patient.

The capacity to use enactments involves 3 components:

- Detect the presence of enactment,
- Analyze its meaning, and
- Use what is learned.

Ultimately, the best protection against destructive enactments, in therapy, but also in other kinds of clinical work with difficult patients, is (1) to have the experience of a personal analysis or therapy to learn one's hooks and blind spots, (2) supervision or consultation, (3) careful negotiation of a therapeutic alliance that includes exploration of what unfolds in the treatment relationship (whether or not it involves therapy), and (4) developing the capacity to "take" the transference that is offered from a stance of warm, empathic, nonjudgmental technical neutrality.

> The best protection against destructive enactments:
>
> - Personal analysis or therapy,
> - Supervision or consultation,
> - Negotiate a therapeutic alliance that includes exploration of the treatment relationship, and
> - Develop the capacity to "take" the transference from a stance of warm, empathic, nonjudgmental technical neutrality.

SUMMARY

There will always be difficult patients, but we are wise to recognize the role we play as individuals and as a profession in contributing to their creation. The biomedical model has not lived up to its promise, but it is currently entrenched in our scientific culture as a relevant "big idea" for the field. The biopsychosocial model is more fully supported by emerging science than is the biomedical model, with "gene-by-environment interaction" just another way of saying "biopsychosocial."

At the level of individual work with patients, we are wise to learn to use psychodynamic concepts like projective identification and enactment to help us understand how we unwittingly co-create the so-called difficult patient.

REFERENCES

1. Plakun EM. Treatment resistance and psychodynamic psychiatry: concepts psychiatry needs from psychoanalysis. Psychodyn Psychiatry 2012;40(2):183–209.
2. Plakun EM, editor. Treatment resistance and patient authority: the Austen Riggs reader. New York: Norton Professional Books; 2011.
3. Box GEP. Science and statistics. J Am Stat Assoc 1976;71:791–9.
4. Engel GL. The need for a new medical model: a challenge for biomedicine. Science 1977;196(4286):129–36.
5. Ghaemi N. On depression: drugs, diagnosis and despair in the modern world. Baltimore (MD): Johns Hopkins; 2013.
6. Collins FS. Shattuck lecture—medical and societal consequences of the Human Genome Project. N Engl J Med 1999;341(1):28–37.
7. Hyde CL, Nagle MW, Tian C, et al. Identification of 15 genetic loci associated with risk of major depression in individuals of European descent. Nat Genet 2016. https://doi.org/10.1038/ng.3623.
8. Cross-Disorder Group of the Psychiatric Genomics Consortium. Identification of risk loci with shared effects on five major psychiatric disorders: a genome-wide analysis. Lancet 2013;381(9875):1371–9.
9. Sekar A, Biala AR, de Rivera H, et al. Schizophrenia risk from complex variation of complement component 4. Nature 2016. https://doi.org/10.1038/nature16549.

10. Kirov G, Pocklington AJ, Holmans P, et al. De novo CNV analysis implicates specific abnormalities of postsynaptic signaling complexes in the pathogenesis of schizophrenia. Mol Psychiatry 2012;17:142–53.
11. Tully EC, Iacono WG, McGue M. An adoption study of parental depression as an environmental liability for adolescent depression and childhood disruptive disorders. Am J Psychiatry 2008;165(9):1148–54.
12. Eley TC, McAdams TA, Rijsdijk FV, et al. The intergenerational transmission of anxiety: a children-of-twins study. Am J Psychiatry 2015;172(7):630–7.
13. Kendler KS, Bulik CM, Silberg J, et al. Childhood sexual abuse and adult psychiatric and substance use disorders in women: an epidemiological and co-twin control analysis. Arch Gen Psychiatry 2000;57:953–9.
14. Molnar BE, Buka SL, Kessler RC. Child sexual abuse and subsequent results from the National Comorbidity Survey. Am J Public Health 2001;91(5):753–60.
15. Joyner MJ, Paneth N, Ioannidis JPA. Viewpoint: what happens when underperforming big ideas in research become entrenched? JAMA 2016;316(13):1355–6.
16. Wisniewski SR, Rush AJ, Nierenberg AA, et al. Can phase III trial results of antidepressant medications be generalized to clinical practice? A STAR*D report. Am J Psychiatry 2009;166:599–607.
17. Skodol AE, Gunderson JG, Shea MT, et al. The Collaborative Longitudinal Personality Disorders Study (CLPS): overview and implications. J Personal Disord 2005; 19:487–504.
18. Bender DS, Skodol AE, Pagano ME, et al. Prospective assessment of treatment use by patients with personality disorders. Psychiatr Serv 2006;57(2):254–7.
19. Skodol AE, Grilo CM, Keyes K, et al. Relationship of personality disorders to the course of major depressive disorder in a nationally representative sample. Am J Psychiatry 2011;168(3):257–64.
20. Caspi A, Houts RM, Belsky DW, et al. The p factor: one general psychopathology factor in the structure of psychiatric disorders? Clin Psychol Sci 2014;2(2): 119–37.
21. Turner EH, Matthews AM, Linardatos E, et al. Selective publication of antidepressant trials and its influence on apparent efficacy. N Engl J Med 2008;358(3): 252–60.
22. Kirsch I, Deacon BJ, Huedo-Medina TB, et al. Initial severity and antidepressant benefits: a meta-analysis of data submitted to the Food and Drug Administration. PLoS Med 2008;5(2):e45.
23. Lieberman JA, Stroup TS, McEvoy JP, et al, Clinical Antipsychotic Trials of Intervention Effectiveness (CATIE) Investigators. Effectiveness of antipsychotic drugs in patients with chronic schizophrenia. N Engl J Med 2005;353:1209–23.
24. Perlis RH, Ostacher MJ, Patel JK, et al. Predictors of recurrence in bipolar disorder: primary outcomes from the Systematic Treatment Enhancement Program for Bipolar Disorder (STEP-BD). Am J Psychiatry 2006;163:217–24.
25. Steinert C, Munder T, Rabung S, et al. Psychodynamic therapy: as efficacious as other empirically supported treatments? A meta-analysis testing equivalence of outcomes. Am J Psychiatry 2017;174(10):943–53.
26. Gilboa-Schechtman E, Foa EB, Shafran N, et al. Prolonged exposure versus dynamic therapy for adolescent PTSD: a pilot randomized controlled trial. J Am Acad Child Adolesc Psychiatry 2010;49:1034–42.
27. Barlow DH, Farchione TJ, Bullis JR, et al. The Unified Protocol for transdiagnostic treatment of emotional disorders compared with diagnosis-specific protocols for anxiety disorders: a randomized clinical trial. JAMA Psychiatry 2017;74(9): 875–84.

28. Johan M. Report of the panel on enactments in psychoanalysis. J Am Psychoanal Assoc 1992;40:827–41.
29. Plakun EM. Sexual misconduct and enactment. J Psychother Pract Res 1999;8: 284–91.
30. Plakun EM. Perspectives on embodiment: from symptom to enactment and from enactment to sexual misconduct. In: Muller JP, Tillman JG, editors. The embodied subject: minding the body in psychoanalysis. Lanham (MD): Rowman and Littlefield; 2007. p. 103–16.
31. Plakun EM. Enactment and the treatment of abuse survivors. Harv Rev Psychiatry 1998;5:318–25.

Treatment-Resistant Depression

The Importance of Identifying and Treating Co-occurring Personality Disorders

Michael Young, MD, MS

KEYWORDS

- Depression • Treatment-resistant depression • Personality traits
- Personality disorder • Borderline personality disorder

KEY POINTS

- Treatment-resistant depression (TRD) is common and produces significant burden to individuals and society. Comprehensive and individualized approaches are needed to address this complex clinical situation.
- Diagnostic reevaluation is indicated in cases of TRD to determine the numerous factors that could be playing a role in the treatment resistance.
- Diagnostic reevaluation in the setting of TRD should include assessment for personality disorders, because these are common contributors to treatment resistance and are often not adequately addressed.
- There are validated psychotherapeutic interventions that have proved effective in treating personality disorders to help patients improve both self-functioning and interpersonal functioning.

INTRODUCTION

Treatment-resistant depression (TRD) is a significant burden to individual patients and society because many individuals with depression do not achieve or sustain remission, despite multiple pharmacologic interventions and treatment settings. Review of the literature reveals many approaches to addressing TRD, including augmentation of antidepressants with atypical antipsychotics and other medications, aerobic exercise, manual-based psychotherapies, and a variety of neurostimulation strategies.[1] Despite this variety of treatment approaches, TRD remains a common and burdensome condition, and each case of TRD requires a thoughtful and individualized treatment approach with attention to the biological, psychological, medical, social, cultural, and spiritual factors involved.

Disclosure: The author has no disclosures.
Sheppard Pratt Health System, 6501 North Charles Street, Towson, MD 21204, USA
E-mail address: myoung@sheppardpratt.org

Psychiatr Clin N Am 41 (2018) 249–261
https://doi.org/10.1016/j.psc.2018.01.003
psych.theclinics.com
0193-953X/18/

Reevaluating the Diagnosis in Treatment-Resistant Depression

TRD often has multiple contributing factors that need to be identified so that they can be addressed with a comprehensive and individualized treatment plan. Reevaluating the clinical diagnoses to help clarify the contributing causes of treatment resistance is an essential component in the assessment of patients with TRD. Common causes of treatment resistance can include misdiagnosis of bipolar depression as unipolar depression, co-occurring substance use disorders, untreated medical conditions, cognitive impairments, trauma disorders, and co-occurring personality disorders. Considering all of these factors in a methodical and thoughtful way is essential in the diagnostic assessment of patients with TRD (**Fig. 1**).

Many psychiatrists have observed treatment resistance resulting from cases in which bipolar depression or mixed states of bipolar disorder have not been recognized and the symptoms have been treated as a unipolar depression. In these cases, the medication regimen often has included antidepressants indicated to treat major depressive disorder but not bipolar disorder. Antidepressants in the setting of bipolar disorder are often ineffective and can potentially exacerbate the symptoms of the bipolar illness and lead to agitation, restlessness, and increased anxiety. Considering the possibility of an underlying bipolar disorder in these cases is often the key to achieving a more effective pharmacologic approach.

In other cases of TRD, there is an underlying substance use disorder (eg, alcohol abuse), untreated or undertreated medical condition (eg, hypothyroidism, cardiovascular disease), underlying cognitive impairment (eg, mild cognitive impairment, dementia), or underlying trauma disorder (eg, posttraumatic stress disorder) complicating or confounding the successful treatment of the depressive episode. Careful history taking, physical examination, urine drug screens, basic medical screening laboratory tests, neurocognitive testing, and brain imaging can often be useful in identifying these contributors of treatment resistance so that appropriate interventions for these complicating factors can be recommended.

In addition to the aforementioned contributors to TRD, co-occurring personality disorders, including a poorly integrated or disrupted sense of self, can contribute significantly to treatment resistance and enduring depressive symptoms. For example, in an avoidant personality disorder there can be low self-esteem, feelings of inferiority, excessive feelings of shame or inadequacy, preoccupation with and sensitivity to criticism or rejection, avoidance of social activity, lack of energy for engaging in life, and a deficit in the capacity to feel pleasure. As another example, in borderline personality disorder (BPD) there can be a poorly developed or unstable self-image; excessive self-criticism; chronic feelings of emptiness; mood instability; frequent feelings of being down and hopeless; feelings of low self-worth; and thoughts of suicide, including

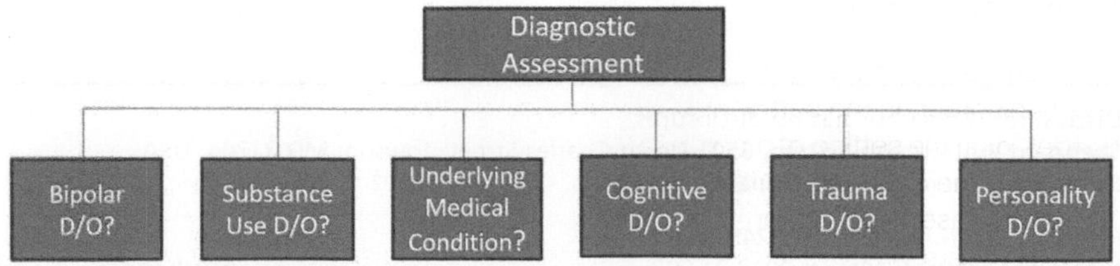

Fig. 1. Diagnostic assessment in TRD. D/O, disorder.

suicidal behavior.[2] It is evident when reviewing the criteria for personality disorders that it can be challenging to distinguish symptoms related to TRD from enduring traits associated with the personality disorder that are fairly stable across time and consistent across different situations. In these cases, the underlying personality structure needs to be addressed specifically as a part of the comprehensive treatment plan if the patient's symptoms are going to be adequately resolved.

Differences in the Quality of Depression with and Without Personality Disorders

Patients with depression and comorbid personality disorders have been shown to differ from patients with depression alone on various measures, including those with personality disorders showing earlier onset, higher severity scores, less social support, more psychosocial stressors, and poorer response to antidepressant medication.[3]

Previous investigators have also examined the relationship of personality traits and disorder to depressive subtype and outcomes in depressed inpatients. It has been reported that personality disorders are more common in unipolar nonmelancholic depressed patients compared with unipolar melancholic or bipolar depressed patients. Furthermore, personality disorder has been related to earlier onset of depressive illness and worse outcome within the unipolar nonmelancholic group of patients. Obsessive traits have been found to be most common in unipolar melancholic patients, whereas histrionic, hostile, and borderline traits have been found to be predominant in nonmelancholic depressed patients.[4] The outcomes described in this study provide additional support for the idea that assessment of personality disorders is an important part of the evaluation in patients with depression, and particularly for patients with a unipolar nonmelancholic subtype of depression.

Further Exploration of Depression Co-occurring with Personality Disorders

The frequent phenomenon of co-occurring depression and personality disorders can be understood from a psychological standpoint by assessing factors that contribute to both depression and personality structure. For example, it has been reported that among types of childhood maltreatment, emotional and physical neglect were the strongest predictors of depression.[5] Because neglectful and inconsistent caregivers during childhood can also contribute to a poorly integrated sense of self that is a hallmark of certain personality disorders, it is sensible that depression and personality disorders can often co-occur in cases in which there is a history of childhood neglect.

As an example of underlying personality disorder complicating the treatment of depression, it has been reported that patients with BPD have a poorer acute response to electroconvulsive therapy.[6] Therefore, one of the gold standards for treating severe and persistent major depressive episodes can be rendered less effective in patients with BPD. In addition, it has been suggested that a diagnosis of BPD has a significant impact on the course of symptoms in self-harming adolescents. Specifically, adolescents with BPD have been shown to have poorer treatment outcomes, including significantly higher levels of clinician-rated and self-reported depressive symptoms and lower levels of global functioning than those without BPD.[7]

TRD can occur in the setting of a biological depression without an underlying personality disorder, in the setting of a biological depression comorbid with a personality disorder, or in the setting of a personality disorder in which the TRD is primarily a manifestation of the enduring traits of the personality disorder (**Fig. 2**).

In some cases, the biological depression can lead to symptoms that appear to others as a personality disorder. This situation can occur when the biological depression, caused by a unipolar or bipolar affective disorder, leads to symptoms such as

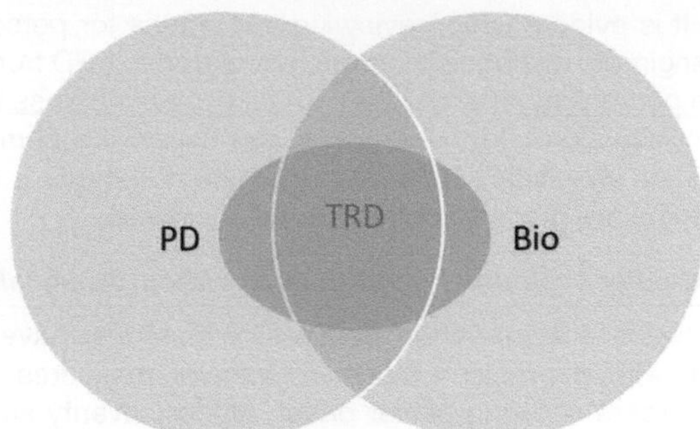

Fig. 2. TRD caused by personality disorder (PD), biological depression (Bio), or a combination.

avoidance, self-criticism, feelings of emptiness, and suicidal behavior, which are common in personality disorders. In these cases, the treatment of the depression and the pseudo–personality disorder is often a biological intervention (eg, medication, neurostimulation) with adjunctive psychotherapeutic intervention (**Fig. 3**). The ability for biological treatment of depression to seemingly alter personality characteristics, such as self-confidence, has also been well described.[8]

In contrast, in some cases, the personality disorder can be the primary cause of persistent depressive symptoms and impairment in social and occupational functioning. In these cases, the primary treatment needed is psychotherapy to address the personality disorder, with the possibility of adding an adjunctive biological intervention (**Fig. 4**). Given the inadequacy of biological interventions alone in treating the persistent depressive symptoms caused by a personality disorder, specific treatment of the personality disorder is indicated. Therefore, it is important for an assessment of personality functioning to take place during the initial assessment and during ongoing follow-up assessments.

Multiple investigators have described the interplay between affective disorders and personality disorders, with a large body of research dealing specifically with connections between affective disorders and BPD. In generally considering the effects of personality disorders on functioning and well-being in the setting of major depressive

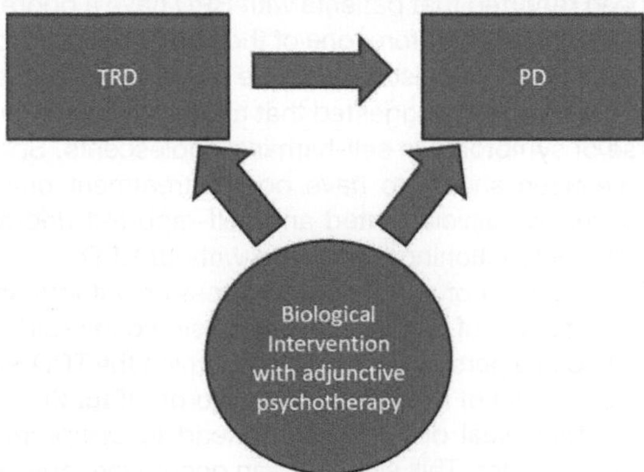

Fig. 3. TRD resulting in PD diagnosis.

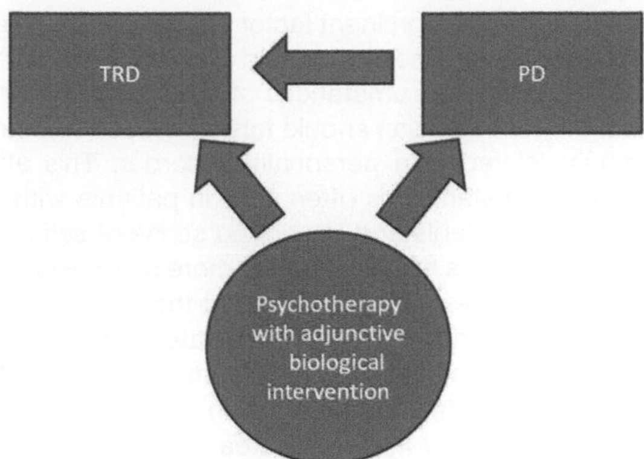

Fig. 4. PD resulting in presentation of TRD.

disorder (MDD), it has been shown that co-occurring personality disorders contribute to impairments in both social and emotional functioning and also decreased sense of well-being.[9] Furthermore, personality disorders at baseline have been shown to predict accelerated relapse after an episode of major depression.[10]

Gunderson and colleagues[11] have done extensive research on the longitudinal course in personality disorders. It has been reported that the course of BPD is characterized by high rates of remission, low rates of relapse, and also severe and persistent impairments in social functioning. This finding points to the importance of identifying and treating co-occurring personality disorders when they occur, so as to improve the social and occupational functioning for patients recovering from depression. This improvement in social and occupational functioning can also be an important factor leading to the patients' recovery from depression.

Gunderson and colleagues[12] also evaluated the interactions of BPD and mood disorders over a 10-year period showing that BPD and MDD showed strong reciprocal effects, delaying each disorder's time to remission and accelerating time to relapse.

Galione and Zimmerman[13] compared depressed patients with and without personality disorder. Depressed patients with personality disorder had a younger age of onset; more depressive episodes; greater likelihood of atypical symptoms; and a higher prevalence of comorbid anxiety disorders, substance use disorders, and number of previous suicide attempts.

Zimmerman and colleagues[14] set out to distinguish bipolar II depression from MDD with comorbid BPD. It was shown that patients with MDD comorbid with BPD were more often diagnosed with posttraumatic stress disorder, current substance use disorder, somatoform disorder, and other nonborderline personality disorders, whereas clinical ratings of anger, anxiety, paranoid ideation, and somatization were significantly higher. It was also reported that the patients with MDD comorbid with BPD were rated lower on the Global Assessment of Functioning scale, had poorer current social functioning, and made significantly more suicide attempts.

Additional Factors in the Diagnostic Assessment for Personality Disorders

To determine the possible contribution of a personality disorder to TRD, a careful diagnostic interview needs to be conducted, with particular focus on the quality of the patient's relationships and on the amount of integration present in the patient's sense of self and others. By including a focus on underlying personality structure and interpersonal functioning during the assessment, clinicians are more likely to identify cases in which personality disorders are a prominent factor in perpetuating the depression. For example, when the patient's depressed mood and comorbid symptoms are highly variable depending on the specific circumstances of the moment or in response to an interpersonal conflict, then the clinician should further assess whether the depressive symptoms are primarily related to a personality disorder. This affective instability based on the external circumstances is often seen in patients with a borderline personality structure, who lack a stable and integrated sense of self and others.

It has been shown that patients with BPD show more self-criticism than depressed patients without BPD.[15] It has also been shown that the psychological constructs of emptiness and abandonment fears are highly associated with borderline disorders.[16] Therefore, the occurrence of these psychological constructs should trigger a more in-depth assessment for BPD as a factor complicating the clinical picture.

A history of self-harm is another important area of assessment in patients being assessed for depression, because self-harm is related to lower levels of global functioning, higher severity of depressive symptoms, and higher levels of self-reported emotional dysregulation.[17] Because self-harm is a common symptom in BPD, this history being present indicates a clear need to assess the personality structure of patients who have self-harmed so that an appropriate intervention can be recommended.

Previous investigators have proposed that a comprehensive clinical assessment combines both an assessment of symptoms and also an assessment of identity, level of defense mechanisms, and global reality testing with a focus on internal representations of self, others, and relationship patterns. The diagnosis of a borderline personality organization and moderate to severe symptoms has been reported to indicate the need for a validated treatment of BPD.[18]

Consideration of Treatment Options for Personality Disorders

An examination of 3 treatments for BPD (dialectical behavioral therapy [DBT], transference-focused psychotherapy, and dynamic supportive treatment) showed that patients in all 3 treatment groups showed significant positive change in depression, anxiety, global functioning, and social adjustment across 1 year of treatment.[19] DBT has been shown to be useful in addressing high suicide risk in individuals with BPD.[20] General psychiatric management (GPM) for patients with BPD is another paradigm developed as an outpatient intervention that can be delivered by independent community health professionals.[21] GPM can be particularly useful if more resource-intensive services such as DBT programs are not available. Mentalization-based therapy (MBT) provides another empirically supported approach to BPD that could be considered.[22]

Case Studies

To show how TRD can be approached by addressing the underlying personality structure of the patient, selected aspects of 2 cases are briefly described here. Characteristics that could identify specific patients have been changed so that confidentiality is maintained.

Mr G: finding a voice

Mr G, a 50-year-old, separated manager of a transportation company, presented to the psychiatric clinic reporting a chronically depressed mood throughout his adulthood and a persistent inability to discuss his emotions and needs with other people. Biological intervention in other settings had not been effective at relieving his depression or in providing relief to his constant feelings of guilt, self-criticism, and passivity.

When asked what he would like help with he replied, "I want to be able to tell other people how I feel without becoming emotional."

Mr G was financially supporting his girlfriend, several of her family members, his adult children, and his ex-wife, despite her having another significant other and a separate life. He was working more than 80 h/wk as a manager of a transportation company to make enough money to support these multiple households financially. He stated that he frequently berates himself for sleeping in on the weekends and feels guilty about not getting more done around the house when he was off from work over the weekend. He described that he has not had the desire to ride his motorcycle like he used to and he becomes guilty when he sees it. He reported that he feels "used" and does not tell people what he wants. He added that he would like to be divorced from his wife and free from paying her mortgage, but he is unable to ask for a divorce, stating, "It's easier to not deal with it...everybody is in control of everything but me...I don't think I'll ever achieve happiness unless I can tell people what I want." He frequently returned to the theme that he is a "doormat." It was evident that at both work and home there was a consistent pattern of him seeing himself as a doormat across multiple domains in his life and with many different people. He described feeling "stuck" in his current circumstances.

When asked about this pattern of being a doormat for others and not being able to assert himself, he was able to describe that his passive nature may be an effort to be "the opposite" of his father. It was noted that his desire to not be like his father was serving to keep him emotionally connected with his father nonetheless.

Mr G's parents divorced when he was 11 years old. His father was harsh, excessively punitive, and frequently told him, "You can do nothing right." After the divorce of his parents, Mr G and his 2 younger siblings were moved around to various apartments in dangerous neighborhoods because of the financial strain of his father's absence. Mr G acknowledged that his inability to ask for a divorce after 9 years could be a demonstration of trying to be the opposite of his father.

Mr G arrived to one session upset about a work meeting earlier in the day; however, he was passive during the meeting and did not advocate for himself. He described, "My feelings won't be perceived well...they'll say I'm negative...they'll say I have to go...the person running the meeting doesn't like me...I get belittled all the time by people who don't know what they are talking about...I feel dismissed and belittled...I checked out...I can't debate it, because I'm never going to win." When asked to imagine how the situation would have played out if he had responded more assertively he replied, "They'd be angry." It was evident that he was experiencing his boss at work as unfairly dismissive and belittling, similar to the way he experienced his father as a child, when self-advocacy or expression of anger was not an option for him.

The inability for Mr G to express anger, even when appropriate, and his inability to advocate for his own needs were identified as central themes that were keeping Mr G in a constant state of despair and feeling put on by others. It was clear that his anger was defended against by his becoming passive and, in his words, a doormat. By identifying this pattern and consistently commenting on this defense to Mr G during sessions, his ability to express anger in the sessions slowly increased.

There were several instances during his therapy during which Mr G developed a significant amount of anger showing up in the transference. One such example was on display during a discussion around a missed appointment, which he initially explained by his statement, "Sometimes I forget things." At the suggestion that his missed appointment could be an unconscious response to the challenge of being in therapy, he became visibly angry during the session and then missed the next session. The following session began with Mr G discussing his irritation that his girlfriend was frequently forgetting things. When asked if this comment could be a masked expression of his irritation at himself for forgetting his last appointment, he became angry and stated, "I never forget anything. I didn't forget my last appointment. I went home and fell asleep and didn't wake up."

Several more months of providing a holding environment for Mr G to become more comfortable expressing his anger enabled Mr G to see that it is possible to express anger and other emotions without destroying himself or others in the process. The shame and guilt associated with his anger lessened, and he came to realize that appropriate expression of anger was an expected and appropriate human behavior. This progress was demonstrated in session when he described his "mini-breakthrough," during which he was able to advocate for himself in a situation with a coworker in which he previously would have remained silent, resented the situation, and directed his anger inward.

Once free to express his wishes and advocate more readily for himself, Mr G no longer was bound to be a doormat for others, which had been leading to a negative view of himself and frequent resentment toward others. He was no longer as burdened by the weight of the world, and he was freer to pursue happiness in his life.

Ms S: finding the self-compassion within

Ms S, a 55-year-old, twice divorced customer service representative, presented to the clinic to undergo treatment of her chronic depression, obsessive compulsive behaviors, attentional difficulties, and anxiety. Ms S described that her chronic depression was frequently severe and caused significant impairment in her social and occupational functioning. Her chronic symptoms included depressed mood, anhedonia, hypersomnia, decreased interest in the world, excessive guilt, low energy, poor concentration, poor appetite, and feeling "disconnected" from her family and friends. On initial presentation she reported various current stressors, including a job she disliked and found unfulfilling, significant financial difficulties, and fear of foreclosure on her home, which was in disrepair and almost uninhabitable because of her hoarding. She described feeling like, "My very presence is an embarrassment," and that she has felt this way for years.

Ms S described enduring many medication trials in the past to help manage her depression; however, she had been exquisitely sensitive to side effects with most medications that were tried. She had been treated with an array of selective serotonin reuptake inhibitors, serotonin-norepinephrine reuptake inhibitors, mood stabilizers, and antipsychotic medications to no avail. She described a particularly bad experience with lithium when she ended up hospitalized because of adverse effects of the medication.

Early in the course of therapy, Ms S's notable masochistic traits became evident. One example of this was seen in her compliant acceptance of a job that she found humiliating and painful coupled with an unwillingness to seek another position. She would frequently describe the horrible work conditions, lack of training opportunities, and unsupportive management that she contended with. Despite having a college degree in education and a history of competent performance working in the insurance industry, she resigned herself to a customer service job in which she felt constantly guilty over not being able to satisfy her customers in addition to receiving poor treatment from her employers. When queried whether changing jobs was a possibility, she was dismissive, stated that no new jobs are listed in the county, and remained determined to suffer through the day-to-day painful experience of her current job.

Ms S also demonstrated her masochism in her inability to allow herself any modicum of joy. During the period surrounding her daughter's wedding, Ms S expressed significant depressed feelings, disconnection, and guilt, stating, "I feel like [my daughter] is leaving me and it is not fair to feel that way…she's entitled to her own life…I feel bad that I'm not happy about her wedding…I can't shake the feeling of sadness…I feel empty inside…I feel very sad and alone…I feel a huge sense of loss…her getting married is the beginning of me having to face the mess I've created for myself."

Another example of Ms S's inability to allow herself to experience positive emotion showed up when she received positive feedback at work, noting her development of an effective working relationship with staff at another location, which was improving customer service. After relating this positive feedback she continued, "Nothing is different…I'm tired, discouraged, disappointed at myself…discouraged at life in general…work isn't any better…I feel like I'm not pulling my weight just like I feel in the rest of my life…it's another environment where I haven't lived up to my capabilities…every second the rug can be pulled from under me and it would be my fault…I'm just so disappointed in myself…my life wasn't supposed to be like this…I expected more of myself…I feel like a major failure."

Because of the notable and extreme sense of guilt, shame, and self-criticism that Ms S displayed across many different scenarios, this was formulated as an area of central importance. Previous investigators have described that identifying the sources of the masochism, be it parents, culture, religion, or otherwise, is an essential part of treating masochism in that it can help patients gain insight into the motives behind the masochistic thoughts and behaviors.[23]

In this vein, Ms S was encouraged to explore the invalidating and sometimes hostile home environment she experienced as a child. She described, "Growing up, Dad was always mad, and Mom was always sad." She stated that she was the middle child in the household and "tried to please everybody." Although she tried to please her parents, she would frequently feel inadequate in her ability to make things right in her household and this caused her significant distress and guilt. In one session she stated, "With my mom's mental illness and my dad's sternness, I always felt like I had done something to make them unhappy…the thought of disappointing my father scared me to death…I spent my life so my dad wouldn't be mad and my mom wouldn't be unhappy…I feel like I've let everybody down…my mom, my dad, and my daughter." When she lamented in a subsequent session, "I don't have a right to expect to feel good or a right to feel happy because my house is in disarray and my finances are a mess," it was evident that she was continuing to experience the unrelenting guilt over not being able to make things right, similar to what she experienced in childhood.

In another session, Ms S provided another illustrative example of the guilt that she experienced as a young child. She related a story dating to when she was 10 years old when she went for a ride in the car with her father. During the trip her father asked both her and her sister which way he should turn, because both ways led to their destination. She said turn right and her sister said turn left. After her father turned right, the car hit a nail in the road and caused a flat tire that needed to be fixed. Ms S responded at the time with a tremendous amount of guilt and personal responsibility. She described, "I felt responsible…I still feel that sense of responsibility…I feel personally responsible that my life hasn't turned out well…due to my financial indiscretions I have no right to have fun…I walk around my whole life feeling bad because I feel responsible for everything bad that's happened…I should have been able to make it better and to do something so that everybody wouldn't be hurting." Ms S carried with her a strong sense of responsibility for her family's dysfunction growing up, which continued to undermine her sense of worthiness throughout her adulthood.

From the point of identifying the origin of Ms S's harsh and critical inner voice, the therapeutic task included lessening the power that this voice held over her. Over the next several sessions, Ms S was able to explore feelings toward her mother for being unavailable at times because of her mental illness and hospitalizations and at other times becoming angry and yelling at the children. Ms S was able to acknowledge the anger she harbored toward her mother and how her mother's critical voice contributed to her poor self-esteem. In becoming more comfortable with acknowledging her anger toward her mother, Ms S was able to direct less of her anger toward herself through self-criticism, which had been perpetuating her depression and contributing to treatment resistance.

The goal for the therapeutic holding environment for Ms S was to provide the space for her to develop self-compassion as a replacement to her self-criticism. This goal was addressed in therapy by helping Ms S gain insight into her suffering so that she could treat herself with more patience and understanding. Working through many sessions in therapy, Ms S slowly started replacing her self-critical internal voice with an internal voice more nurturing and accepting of imperfection. After several months of working on a more self-compassionate inner voice, Ms S discussed what her daughter wanted for her, stating, "She wants to see me happy and feel successful…to be in a relationship…because she knows I have a lot to give." Ms S was starting to give herself the permission to get well.

Further Discussion of Case Studies

In the case of Mr G, participation in psychotherapy enabled him to achieve significant relief from his depressive symptoms and improvement in both social and occupational functioning. Although the biological intervention of medication management had not been effective, the psychotherapeutic intervention ultimately allowed for relief from the feelings of guilt, self-criticism, and passivity that had limited his capacity to advocate for himself and make decisions in support of his well-being and happiness. During the course of treatment, he developed the capacity to advocate for a more manageable work schedule and request more shared responsibility from those he had been financially supporting so he could achieve a better work-life balance. He also developed a greater capacity to advocate for his own needs in his interpersonal relationships, which he could readily notice and appreciate. This psychological growth in Mr G occurred over approximately 2 years of weekly psychodynamically informed supportive psychotherapy. This type of psychotherapy both reinforces the patient's adaptive coping mechanisms and strengths and provides a safe space to explore the maladaptive defense mechanisms that are present, underlying motivations influencing behavior, and patterns that have developed in interpersonal relationships over time. Focus on the transference, and particularly the anger that presented in the room during sessions, was a very useful technique that allowed Mr G to gain better insight into his own psychological functioning.

Ms S was also able to achieve significant relief from her depressive symptoms and an improvement in functioning as a result of her participation in psychotherapy. Although several medication trials were not adequate to achieve remission of her depression, the psychotherapeutic intervention provided her a framework to allow herself to heal. Similar to the case of Mr G, the personal growth in Ms S occurred over approximately 2 years of weekly psychodynamically informed supportive psychotherapy. Because of a fragile sense of self that often left her feeling dejected and self-critical, a supportive and encouraging therapeutic relationship helped to build a trustworthy foundation for some of the deeper insight-oriented work that occurred later in the course of treatment. Early in the treatment, cognitive behavioral techniques were also used to help Ms S achieve more immediate control of her hoarding behavior, which was contributing to a significant amount of daily stress. Ultimately, a psychodynamic psychotherapy approach, with a focus on how her experiences in childhood have significantly affected her thought patterns, emotions, and behavior throughout her adulthood, proved to be a key element of Ms S's ability to free herself from her compulsive masochism. During the latter part of the treatment, her improvement in social functioning was evident in her positive descriptions of her new role as grandmother and in her reengagement as a positive presence in her daughter's life.

SUMMARY

Although the dual-diagnosis approach of treating 2 disorders simultaneously is frequently discussed in the setting of substance use disorders co-occurring with affective disorders, this dual-diagnosis terminology is not often applied in the setting of personality disorders co-occurring with depression. However, similar to how depression often cannot be effectively treated in the setting of active substance abuse, depression often cannot be effectively treated in the setting of an active personality disorder, unless the personality disorder is addressed in an effective way. Therefore, it would be sensible to adopt the dual-diagnosis approach when a patient is experiencing TRD and a personality disorder is diagnosed or suspected.

Psychotherapy can be particularly useful in managing symptoms of depression and also comorbid symptoms that contribute to treatment resistance, including personality disorders. Acceptance and commitment treatment, cognitive behavioral analysis system of psychotherapy, DBT, and mindfulness-based cognitive therapy have all shown evidence for treatment of TRD.[24] Current evidence also supports the efficacy of psychodynamic psychotherapy. A review of the effectiveness of psychodynamic psychotherapy has shown a trend toward larger effect sizes at follow-up, indicating continued improvement in symptoms after the course of therapy has ended.[25]

Given that there are now multiple validated methods for treating various personality disorders, psychotherapy to address underlying personality disorders should be considered as a first-line, standard-of-care approach in the setting of TRD when there is a personality disorder diagnosed or suspected.

Reasons that have been given to explain the difficulty in treating comorbid personality disorders include the significant time commitment that treatment requires, a shortage of clinicians trained in treating personality disorders, and the presumed high cost of effective treatment. However, given the exceedingly high costs of TRD to both individuals and society, it is essential for clinicians to recognize the significant role that personality disorders can play in TRD and recommend a treatment plan to address the personality disorders when present. Given the long-recognized observation by clinical psychotherapists and the emerging research evidence that personality disorders can be effectively treated, a strong case can be made that investing resources into treatment of personality disorders must be a priority in modern psychiatry.

In the case examples described earlier, it was the psychotherapeutic intervention of providing a safe and supportive holding environment to foster the development of greater insight and self-compassion that enabled Mr G and Ms S to gain traction in their journeys of recovery.

ACKNOWLEDGMENTS

The author would like to thank Dr Don Ross, MD, a psychiatrist in the Sheppard Pratt Health System and faculty at the University of Maryland/Sheppard Pratt Psychiatry Residency Program, for his assistance with this article.

REFERENCES

1. McIntyre R, Filteau M, Martin L, et al. Treatment-resistant depression: definitions, review of the evidence, and algorithmic approach. J Affect Disord 2014;156:1–7.
2. Diagnostic and statistical manual of mental disorders: DSM-5. 5th edition. Arlington (VA): American Psychiatric Association; 2013. p. 645–84.
3. Pfohl B, Stangl D, Zimmerman M. The implications of DSM-III personality disorders for patients with major depression. J Affect Disord 1984;7:309–18.
4. Charney D, Nelson C, Quinlan D. Personality traits and disorder in depression. Am J Psychiatry 1981;138:1601–4.
5. Liu J, Gong J, Nie G, et al. The mediating effects of childhood neglect on the association between schizotypal and autistic personality traits and depression in a non-clinical sample. BMC Psychiatry 2017;17:352.
6. Feske U, Mulsant B, Pilkonis P, et al. Clinical outcome of ECT in patients with major depression and comorbid borderline personality disorder. Am J Psychiatry 2004;161:2073–80.
7. Ramleth R, Groholt B, Diep L, et al. The impact of borderline personality disorder and sub-threshold borderline personality disorder on the course of self-reported and clinician-rated depression in self-harming adolescents. Borderline Personal Disord Emot Dysregul 2017;4:22.
8. Kramer P. Listening to Prozac. Makeover. New York: Penguin Books; 1993. p. 1–21.
9. Skodol A, Grilo C, Pagano M, et al. Effects of personality disorders on functioning and well-being in major depressive disorder. J Psychiatr Pract 2005;11:363–8.
10. Grilo C, Stout R, Markowitz J, et al. Personality disorders predict relapse after remission from an episode of major depressive disorder: a 6-year prospective study. J Clin Psychiatry 2010;71:1629–35.
11. Gunderson J, Stout R, McGlashan T, et al. Ten-year course of borderline personality disorder: psychopathology and function from the Collaborative Longitudinal Personality Disorders study. Arch Gen Psychiatry 2011;68:827–37.
12. Gunderson J, Stout R, Shea M, et al. Interactions of borderline personality disorder and mood disorders over 10 years. J Clin Psychiatry 2014;75:829–34.
13. Galione J, Zimmerman M. A comparison of depressed patients with and without borderline personality disorder: implications for interpreting studies of the validity of the bipolar spectrum. J Pers Disord 2010;24:763–72.
14. Zimmerman M, Martinez H, Morgan T, et al. Distinguishing bipolar II depression from major depressive disorder with comorbid borderline personality disorder: demographic, clinical, and family history differences. J Clin Psychiatry 2013;74:880–6.
15. Southwick SM, Yehuda R, Giller EL. Psychological dimensions of depression in borderline personality disorder. Am J Psychiatry 1995;152:789–91.
16. Rogers J, Widiger T, Krupp A. Aspects of depression associated with borderline personality disorder. Am J Psychiatry 1995;152:268–70.
17. Weintraub M, Van de Loo M, Gitlin M, et al. Self-harm, affective traits, and psychosocial functioning in adults with depressive and bipolar disorders. J Nerv Ment Dis 2017;205:896–9.
18. Yeomans F, Clarkin J, Kernberg O. Transference-focused psychotherapy for borderline personality disorder: a clinical guide. In: Assessment phase: clinical evaluation and treatment selection. Washington, DC: American Psychiatric Publishing; 2015. p. 83–98.
19. Clarkin J, Levy K, Lenzenweger M, et al. Evaluating three treatments for borderline personality disorder: a multiwave study. Am J Psychiatry 2007;164:922–8.

20. Linehan M, Korslund K, Harned M, et al. Dialectical behavior therapy for high suicide risk in individuals with borderline personality disorder: a randomized clinical trial and component analysis. JAMA Psychiatry 2015;72:475–82.
21. Links P, Ross J, Gunderson J. Promoting good psychiatric management for patients with borderline personality disorder. J Clin Psychol 2015;71:753–63.
22. Daubney M, Bateman A. Mentalization-based therapy (MBT): an overview. Australas Psychiatry 2015;23:132–5.
23. Hailparn D, Hailparn M. The song of the siren: dealing with masochistic thoughts and behaviors. J Contemp Psychother 2004;34:163–80.
24. Moukaddam N, Hashmi A, Nguyen P. Use of psychotherapy in treatment-resistant depression. Psychiatr Ann 2016;46:230–5.
25. Shedler J. The efficacy of psychodynamic psychotherapy. Am Psychol 2010;65:98–109.

The Overall Diagnosis

Psychodynamic Psychiatry, Six-Minute Psychotherapy, and Patient-Centered Care

Elizabeth Weinberg, MD*, David Mintz, MD

KEYWORDS

- Psychodynamic psychopharmacology • Patient-centered medicine • Alliance
- Psychotherapy

KEY POINTS

- Patient-centered medicine derives from the work of Michael and Enid Balint, and provides a path by which psychiatry can reengage psychodynamic concepts to improve patient care.
- Key concepts in patient-centered medicine include the biopsychosocial perspective, the patient-as-person, the doctor-as-person, shared responsibility and authority, and the therapeutic alliance.
- Corresponding principles in psychodynamic psychiatry support the development of the treatment relationship and improved outcomes in psychiatric treatment.
- The prescribing psychiatrist can use a modified form of psychodynamic psychotherapy to enhance patient care.

We physicians cannot discard psychotherapy, if only because another person intimately concerned in the process of recovery —the patient—has no intention of discarding it... A factor dependent on the psychical disposition of the patient contributes, without any intention on our part, to the effect of every therapeutic process initiated by a physician; most frequently it is favorable to recovery, but often it acts as an inhibition.... All physicians, therefore, yourselves included, are continually practicing psychotherapy, even when you have no intention of doing so and are not aware of it.

—Freud, S. (1905). On Psychotherapy, p. 258–259

INTRODUCTION

The explosion of knowledge owing to biological research in psychiatry has been accompanied by decreased emphasis on psychological understanding of patients,

---

Disclosure Statement: No financial interests to disclose.

Austen Riggs Center, 25 Main Street, Box 962, Stockbridge, MA 01262, USA
* Corresponding author.
E-mail address: Elizabeth.Weinberg@austenriggs.net

Psychiatr Clin N Am 41 (2018) 263–275
https://doi.org/10.1016/j.psc.2018.01.008
psych.theclinics.com

their illnesses, and the treatment relationship. Meanwhile, the development of patient-centered medicine[1] has led to an increased appreciation in primary care of nonbiologic dimensions of care. Patient-centered medicine, developed from the work of the psychoanalytic theorist Michael Balint, has its roots in psychodynamic concepts. These concepts can assist the prescribing psychiatrist in better understanding the patient's needs, improving the therapeutic alliance, and integrating modified psychotherapy.

PSYCHIATRY IN THE AGE OF NEUROSCIENCE

The excitement accompanying the great research discoveries in biological psychiatry during the last century[2] was accompanied by pressure on physicians to focus on biological interventions. Pharmacotherapy in general is better compensated than psychotherapy, and American publishing has shifted from favoring the psychological to focusing on psychopharmacologic research.[3] Meanwhile, as psychiatry has become increasingly focused on the medical model, general medicine experienced an upsurge of interest in patient-centered care, bringing a focus to the "patient-as-person" and "doctor-as-person" to the practice of medicine.[4] Tellingly, in 1 metaanalysis,[5] out of 26 studies examining the effects of psychosocial interventions to improve antidepressant adherence, 25 came from the primary care literature and only 1 from organized psychiatry.

In 2010, then director of the National Institutes of Mental Health Thomas Insell[6] wrote in explaining the purpose of the Research Domain Criteria (RDoC) project that guides National Institutes of Mental Health funding, that the RDoC assumes that mental illnesses are best conceptualized as brain disorders, that the corresponding dysfunction of brain circuits could be identified using tools of clinical neuroscience, and that data from neuroscience would yield "biosignatures" that would lead to improved clinical management. In 2017, in an interview for *Wired* magazine,[7] Insell admitted that 13 years of neuroscientific research had not "moved the needle" in addressing suicide, hospitalizations, or psychiatric recovery.

Our field has invested much of its creativity and resources in biomedical research. Meanwhile, rates of death by suicide have increased significantly since 2000,[8] outcomes of treatment for serious mental illness are not notably improved, and treatment resistance has become increasingly prominent in the psychiatric literature.[9] One likely reason that neuroscientific advances seem not to have transformed the experience of real-world patients is that psychiatry has neglected some of its most potent tools. In allowing itself to be increasingly restricted to biomedical targets, the field neglected the profound influence of psychosocial interventions on treatment outcomes.

PSYCHODYNAMICS AND THE ORIGINS OF PATIENT-CENTERED CARE

In 1930, the physician, psychoanalyst, and progenitor of patient-centered medicine, Michael Balint, noted the growth of pharmacologic advertising and laboratory tests. He observed concordant changes in practice. Older physicians, he noted, were skilled in sensitive clinical observation,[10] whereas younger physicians seemed to know their patients less well. Although Balint wrote nearly 90 years ago, his observations seem applicable to our own experience. Balint's work became the basis for the movement known as patient-centered medicine, a term he coined in his work with his collaborator and spouse, Enid Balint.[11,12] The Balints advocated for the concept of the "overall diagnosis."[13] "This should include everything that the doctor know and understands about his patient; the patient, in fact, has to be understood as a unique human being."[12]

The Institute of Medicine,[14] in an influential report, designated patient-centered care as 1 of the 6 priorities for development of health care systems for the 21st century. In 2013, an editorial in *Psychiatric News* announced that psychiatry as field was ready to embrace patient-centered care.[15] It is an irony of psychiatric practice that although the concept of patient-centered medicine emerged from psychodynamic psychiatry, psychiatry now lags general medicine in attunement to the values of patient-centered medicine.

PATIENT-CENTERED MEDICINE AND PSYCHODYNAMIC PSYCHIATRY

Mead and Bower,[4] in their highly cited paper, identified 5 conceptual dimensions to patient-centered care. These include:

1. The biopsychosocial perspective,
2. Awareness of the "patient-as-person,"
3. Shared responsibility and authority between doctor and patient,
4. A focus on the therapeutic alliance, and
5. Awareness of the "doctor-as-person."

The psychoanalytic roots of these dimensions appear clearly in Michael Balint's 1957 text on the use of psychotherapeutic technique in medical practice.[16] Balint theorized that medical complaints could be connected to underlying psychological vulnerabilities he called "the basic fault."[16,17] Balint believed that often the patient's difficulties related to the fundamental need for love, and observed that the act of making a medical complaint has emotional, social, and interpersonal meaning.

Balint regarded a thorough assessment as particularly important in the treatment of "fat envelope" patients,[16] that is, those patients who often used the medical system, resulting in voluminous medical charts. He initiated the use of "Balint groups," in which physicians could support each other in psychologically informed work, a type of group still in use in primary care, and trained physicians in "six minute psychotherapy,"[12] in which physicians could provide limited therapy in medical practice. At the time that the Balints were seeking to help primary care providers develop basic psychodynamic skills, it would have been inconceivable that psychiatrists would be in need of them. Now, however, it is precisely such skills that are needed by contemporary psychiatrists to restore psychiatry to a balanced, integrative position.

There are varying definitions of psychodynamic practice. As Gabbard[18] notes, psychodynamic practice goes beyond therapeutic technique in conveying a "way of thinking" about people that includes interest in the unconscious, in psychological conflict, relationships, and the meanings of lived experience. Blagys and Hilsenroth[19] describe the essential features of psychodynamic treatments: a focus on affect states and emotional expression; exploration of avoidance and resistance to treatment; identification of patterns in thoughts, feelings, and relationships; an emphasis on past experience; focus on interpersonal relationships; an emphasis on the therapeutic relationship; and the exploration of meanings in wishes, dreams, and fantasies.

Academic bias against psychodynamic concepts[20] has led psychodynamic theory to fall out of favor in contemporary psychiatry, despite the proliferation of studies that demonstrate the effectiveness of psychodynamic interventions.[21] Yet, comparing recommendations from patient-centered medicine and psychodynamic treatment models reveals they share commonalities that emerge from the psychodynamic origins of patient-centered medicine (**Table 1**).

The psychodynamic model incorporates and goes beyond the biopsychosocial model by recognizing that the patient's varied concerns, wishes, and goals may be

Table 1
Patient-centered medicine and psychodynamic psychopharmacology

PCM	PP	Clinical Application
Biopsychosocial perspective	Avoid a mind-body split	Understand the impact of psychosocial factors on outcome
Patient as person	Know who the patient is	Understand how the patient's life history and psychology affect healthy use of treatment Psychodynamic formulation
Focus on therapeutic alliance	Cultivate the alliance	Skillful clinical communication Address ways that negative expectations of care undercut treatment effectiveness
Shared responsibility and authority	Attend to the patient's ambivalent wishes	Respect for patient authority Attend to patient preferences and involve patient in shared decision making
Doctor as person	Attend to countertransference	Physician's use of self-reflection Use of psychodynamic formulation to manage countertransference
Patient and doctor as people	Countertherapeutic uses of medication	Detect and address enactments

Abbreviations: PCM, patient-centered medicine; PP, psychodynamic psychopharmacology.

in conflict, and that the patient's ambivalence in the face of such conflict may not be fully conscious. Patients' avoidance of and resistance to treatment can be best addressed when such ambivalence is identified and understood. Similarly, the psychodynamic model goes beyond the precepts of contemporary patient-centered care by recognizing that physicians may also be affected by feelings, motivations, and conflicts outside the range of their awareness. Patients may use medications for reasons that have nothing to do with pharmacologic effectiveness, and physicians may comply in part because of unconscious motivations and anxieties, leading to the countertherapeutic use of medication.[9]

When treatment resistance arises from difficulties at the level of meaning, it can only be addressed at that level. "Psychodynamic psychopharmacology,"[9] born from work with treatment-resistant patients, represents one attempt to develop a psychodynamically informed, patient-centered approach to treatment resistance.

Mintz and Flynn[22] have articulated 6 technical principles:

1. Avoid a mind-body split;
2. Know who the patient is;
3. Attend to ambivalence about loss of symptoms;
4. Cultivate the therapeutic alliance;
5. Attend to countertherapeutic uses of medications; and
6. Identify, contain, and use countertransference.

These principles form the basis of the practice of medical psychotherapy, guided by psychodynamic concepts, that does not require excessive time, and can be incorporated into the routine practice of pharmacotherapy. These principles are also supported by a robust evidence base.[22] Correspondences between the technical principles of psychodynamic psychiatry and patient-centered medicine can be seen in **Table 1**.

THE BIOPSYCHOSOCIAL PERSPECTIVE: HOW TO AVOID A MIND-BODY SPLIT

The medical model of disease posits an identifiable, biologically based source of pathology that can be targeted by a specific medical treatment. Although there are some medical causes of mood disorders in which this model applies, such as thyroid disorders, at present it seems to be most likely that most psychiatric illnesses are multifactorial in origin. The neurobiological model of mental illness in general is a deterministic theory, because it contains the implicit assumption that if everything can be known and understood about the biology underlying mental illness, this can lead to a complete understanding of mental illness itself. Using, however, mathematical observations of the dynamics of complex systems and observations drawn from chaos theory,[23] we can see that, in much of ordinary life, no matter how much we know about the physical conditions at hand, there is far too much complexity and uncertainty for us to predict how 1 action or event will influence others. If this is true of our physical environment, how much more true it is likely to be of the complexities of psychological experience. Furthermore, the philosophic discourse regarding the "hard problem" of consciousness[24] demonstrates that, although it is in principle easy to describe how neurologic processes work in a physical sense, it is not possible for us to extrapolate from this to understand the subjective nature of conscious experience. As much as it may be useful to learn about the brain, we are likely never to be able to understand everything there is to know about the nature of psychological experience by studying the brain alone.

In avoiding a mind-body split, the psychodynamic practitioner acknowledges that in fact all mental illnesses are brain diseases, or at any rate reflect events in the brain, but maintains that this does not substantially differentiate psychiatric illness from experiences, such as reading poetry or falling in love, which also are registered in the brain. Clearly, there are important findings regarding the correlation of brain abnormalities with clinical pathology in psychiatric illnesses. Psychotherapy also changes the brain structurally,[25,26] and has been hypothesized to intervene at the level of gene expression.[27] In refusing to capitulate to Cartesian dualism, psychodynamic psychiatry treats mental illness as a set of human experiences, some of which are strongly influenced by identifiable biological factors, but many of which are more reflective of complex interactions between the body, life experience, and psychological adaptation.

Although genetic research often assumes that psychiatric illnesses are "highly heritable neuropsychiatric" disorders,[28] information accumulates demonstrating contributions of early adversity and environmental stress. Large community samples demonstrate a dose-disease relationship between adverse childhood experiences and general mental health problems,[29] as well as severe medical illnesses.[30] Similarly, a World Health Organization–sponsored study[31] found a strong association between adverse childhood experiences and adult *Diagnostic and Statistical Manual of Mental Disorders,* 4th edition (DSM-IV), psychiatric diagnoses. Psychotic disorders, often assumed to be primarily neuropsychiatric in origin, have been associated with childhood adversity,[32] living in an urban environment,[33] and immigrant status.[34]

Evidence regarding the importance of childhood experiences and social stress in adulthood add complexity to exclusively biological models of psychiatric illness. In 1 neurodevelopmental model of psychosis,[35] long-term social defeat contributes to chronic dopaminergic sensitization and increased baseline activity of the mesolimbic dopamine system. Similarly, Caspi and colleagues[36,37] found that individuals carrying the short allele (S) of the region (*5-HTTLPR*) of the 5-HTT gene were more likely to develop depression when also exposed to childhood maltreatment. They hypothesize that there is a link between the effects of the S allele and a neurologic mechanism that may underlie its effects involving increased reactivity to stress.

Clinically, such findings support the biopsychosocial model,[38] in which biological, psychological, and social influences operate at different levels of organization. Disturbance at any one of these levels is likely to disrupt functioning. At the same time, stabilizing interventions at 1 level can also stabilize the system as a whole. Medical psychotherapy, because of its flexibility, interpersonal responsiveness and attention to the "overall diagnosis" can provide such stabilization.

THE PATIENT-AS-PERSON: KNOW WHO THE PATIENT IS

A sensitive understanding of the patient includes the development of a formulation that addresses relevant historical, psychological, social, and biological factors, consistent with the Balint's concept of the "overall diagnosis."[12] Although the psychodynamic approach does not have a monopoly on the use of complex data in a formulation, the psychodynamic approach is the only one that explicitly includes past, present, interpersonal, affective, and unconscious dimensions. As Perry and associates describe in their classic paper,[39] the aim of the psychodynamic formulation is to guide the treatment and lend it coherence and stability. An effective formulation integrates understanding of the patient's medical problems, personal history, psychological conflicts, and modes of coping with discomfort and anxiety, informing the course of treatment.

Personality styles and pathology[40] influence treatment response. Neuroticism, a personality style characterized by vulnerability to negative affective states, can contribute to poor treatment response to medication[40] and also can increase the patient's experience of side effects.[41] Similarly, an immature defense style predicted poor response to an antidepressant, but not to psychotherapy.[42] Conversely, patients with an internal locus of control may respond more positively to treatment.[43]

Patients' expectations influence the placebo response, arguably contributing to the majority of beneficial effects of some classes of psychotropic medications.[44] Placebo effects of medication can be influenced by diverse factors, including their cost and even their color,[45,46] and in 1 study were doubled with an "enriched" clinical relationship,[47] pointing to the central importance of the clinical relationship in pharmacotherapy.

The inverse of the placebo is the nocebo,[48] that is negative reactions to inactive agents, related to negative expectations or feelings about the medication, as illustrated in Case 1. In 1 trial, researchers found an incidence of roughly 1 in 20 adverse events per prescribed placebo.[49] Nonpharmacologic responses to medication can be connected to unconscious[50] expectations about treatment or about the physician.[51]

Case 1

Lisa is a young woman who presents with chronic anxiety and depression, seeking medication for anxiety and depression. She has experienced intolerable diarrhea with every medication she tried. Review of her history uncovered a pattern of concerns about control and autonomy, including an intrusive, controlling relationship with her mother and experiences of sexual aggression with romantic partners. Lisa and her psychiatrist agreed to meet regularly, make medication changes slowly, and attend carefully to Lisa's reactions. Having formed an alliance that attended to Lisa's needs for control over her bodily functions, she was able to find and tolerate medications that addressed her psychiatric symptoms.

Case example represents condensed versions of cases using disguised, composite clinical details, meant to illustrate the clinical utility of these points without revealing potentially identifying patient information.

THE DOCTOR-AS-PERSON: ATTEND TO COUNTERTRANSFERENCE

If patient characteristics contribute to treatment response, those of the practitioner do as well. McKay and colleagues[52] conducted an analysis of data from the Treatment of Depression Collaborative Research program, comparing relative responses to antidepressant and placebo. This study evaluated variation in treatment response based on prescriber, contrasted with variation owing to drug versus placebo. The authors found that differences of patient response to specific psychiatrists were greater than the differences between the medication and placebo.

As Ankarberg and Falkenström[53] have noted, there has been little attention in psychiatric treatment guidelines to the psychosocial characteristics of psychiatric prescribing, although almost all drug studies occur in the context of active therapeutic engagement with a prescribing physician. Furthermore, pharmaceutical studies that feature limited personal contact with the prescribing physician and study personnel seem to achieve significantly worse results than those with generous contact with prescribers, leading to the observation[53] that the primary active agent in pharmacologic treatment is the interpersonal contact with treaters, not the specific pharmacologic effects of a medication.

Van Os and colleagues[54] identified a dimension of care that they termed "communicative skillfulness," characterized by empathy and supportive interactions. Depressed patients who were treated with depression-specific interventions improved when their physicians showed communicative skillfulness, but worsened when the prescriber had little communicative skill. Interestingly, communicative skillfulness in the absence of a depression-specific intervention was not effective; what was required for effective treatment was the combination of an appropriate intervention with communicative skill.

Although a careful prescriber can recognize the manifestations of problematic countertransference reactions, prescribing that goes against the prescriber's best judgment suggests the physician is acting out unconscious emotional and psychological reactions (Case 2). Identifying and addressing these reactions can restore the safety and effectiveness of the treatment.

Case 2

Joan is a busy mother who repeatedly contacts her psychiatrist with complaints of intolerable stress and requests for relief. Her doctor, who feels both frustrated with Joan's demands and guilty about not being able to provide more lasting relief, starts to provide increasing doses of benzodiazepines. Eventually, Joan's husband calls the doctor, irate that Joan is so sedated and confused that she can barely function.

Case example represents condensed versions of cases using disguised, composite clinical details, meant to illustrate the clinical utility of these points without revealing potentially identifying patient information.

THE TREATMENT RELATIONSHIP AND THE ALLIANCE

The literature on the treatment alliance owes much to psychoanalytic thought. Specific concepts deriving from psychoanalysis include the therapeutic alliance,[55] the working alliance,[56] and the real relationship.[57] If a treatment plan can only be effective when the patient adheres to recommendations, an effective treatment alliance perhaps is the most critical tool in establishing the optimal conditions for treatment response. A truly patient-centered practice hinges on recognizing the patient's subjectivity, and that experiences of illness and treatment are invested with meaning.

Several studies have identified direct correlations between treatment alliance and psychopharmacologic treatment response. Krupnick and colleagues[58] found that remission after treatment of depression with interpersonal psychotherapy, cognitive behavioral therapy, or pharmacotherapy was strongly related to the quality of the treatment alliance. Attention to the treatment alliance both enhances adherence and general treatment response.[59] Aspects of the treatment relationship rated by patients as important to the treatment alliance and that seem to be correlated with treatment response, include patient's perceptions of the clinician as collaborative, compassionate, available, and empathic.[60]

SHARING RESPONSIBILITY IN CLINICAL CARE: ATTENDING TO AMBIVALENCE

Patient-centered medicine places particular emphasis on shared responsibility and authority between doctor and patient. This paradigm reflects a cultural shift away from seeing the patient as the relatively passive recipient of medical care, toward playing an active role in partnership with the physician. As Woolley and colleagues[61] found in a survey of more than 400 patients being treated with antidepressants, discontinuation rates were increased by 7-fold among patients who disagreed with their treatment and felt uninvolved in treatment decisions.

As Gutheil noted,[62] "alliance" may be confused with "compliance." Because of the overtones of passivity implied by the term "compliance," "adherence"[63] increasingly has come into use as a term that describes persistent commitment to following the prescribed treatment plan. Although this term acknowledges the patient's agency, it does not leave room for ambivalence.

A psychodynamic perspective adds to the idea of patient authority the recognition that both patient and doctor make choices influenced by the unconscious. Treatment cannot be effective in the absence of adherence to treatment, and problems in adherence can often not be fully understood and addressed without appreciating the patient's conflicting, ambivalent desires.

A lack of adherence commonly disrupts treatment.[64,65] Reasons for nonadherence are various and complex. In studies examining actual reasons for nonadherence cited by patients, common reasons include perceived poor communication with the prescriber, unwillingness to allow medication to control their emotions, distress at the idea of having a chronic illness, and the experience of problematic side effects.[66,67] Patients may miss or value psychiatric symptoms.[9,66,67] Problems with adherence can only be understood from the patient's point of view, including the reality that the clinician's goals for treatment and view of the illness may not fully coincide with those of the patient.

PATIENT-AS-PERSON MEETS DOCTOR-AS-PERSON: THE PROBLEM OF COUNTERTHERAPEUTIC USES OF MEDICINE

One unintended consequence of the "chemical imbalance" theory of psychiatric illness is that ordinary but unpleasant feelings such as sadness and anger may be stigmatized, medicalized, and stripped of meaning. Moreover, because prescribing has taken the place of psychotherapy, adolescents and young adults may grow up never having experienced emotional reactions and sexual response without mediation and interference by psychiatric medication. George's use of medication, as we see in the case example in Case 3, seems to be influenced by his parents' guilt about the effect of their divorce, his struggle to manage new and confusing feelings of sadness and anger, and his psychiatrist's wish to be helpful. In this kind of case, a psychiatrist who monitors his own reactions and who seeks to understand the patient's developmental needs may be able to do much to offer the patient support and relief, and minimize unnecessary prescribing (Case 3).

Case 3

George is an 18-year-old man who has been on antidepressants since he was 10, when his parents were seeking a divorce and they thought he might be depressed. When George started to argue with his mother at age 16, his parents spoke to his psychiatrist, who prescribed a mood stabilizer. George believes that he has a "chemical imbalance," that makes him prone to irrational depression and anger. Recently, he and his girlfriend started to argue, and he is worried he is getting "sick" because he is feeling sad and angry. He also notes that, at age 18, he almost never has erections or experiences sexual excitement, which he connects with the medications he has taken consistently since before puberty.

Case example represents condensed versions of cases using disguised, composite clinical details, meant to illustrate the clinical utility of these points without revealing potentially identifying patient information.

THE ROLE OF MEDICAL PSYCHOTHERAPY

Too often, discussions of psychiatric treatment have treated psychopharmacology and psychotherapy as though they are mutually exclusive. Huhn and colleagues[68] conducted a review of 852 psychiatric metaanalyses addressing the treatment efficacy of pharmacotherapy or psychotherapy versus placebo, pharmacotherapy versus placebo, and their combination versus either treatment alone. Their findings were that psychotherapy and pharmacotherapy had roughly equal effect sizes, which were assessed as "medium," and that the combination of psychotherapy and pharmacotherapy was more effective than either treatment alone.

Although, increasingly, psychiatrists specialize in the prescription of medication and refer to other clinicians for psychotherapy, it is worth considering the role of psychotherapy as part of routine psychiatric practice. Psychotherapy and psychopharmacology[69] often can be best integrated when offered by the same clinician. Combining psychotherapy and psychopharmacology may be more cost effective and preferred by the patient. Exclusively prescribing psychiatrists also benefit from developing familiarity with medical psychotherapy. The prescribing relationship is inherently subject to transference and countertransference, and the patient and physician must negotiate grounds for trust and communication. Finally, as noted by Freud,[70] however, the physician intends to practice, the patient ultimately is inevitably affected by the therapeutic (or countertherapeutic) nature of the clinical encounter.

Michael and Enid Balint advocated for "six minute psychotherapy"[12] that could be incorporated into the usual appointment. Rather than pursuing grand psychological insights, they suggested much could be accomplished from "little bang" understanding; that patient and physician working together can gradually deepen their understanding of the patient's difficulties in relatively small ways that enhance the cooperative nature of their relationship and clarify the patient's difficulties. Mintz and Belnap's treatment of Psychodynamic Psychopharmacology[9] provides technical to guide prescribers in exploring the meanings of medication and illness, and addressing countertherapeutic forces in the patient and the doctor-patient relationship.

Psychopharmacology, as is true of any aspect of the practice of medicine, is a cooperative, interpersonal endeavor that involves a shared goal of healing and the development of mutual understanding and familiarity. When treatment involves communication, exploration, and a treatment relationship with a shared expectation of healing, it falls within a broad definition of psychotherapy,[71] even without explicit psychotherapeutic goals. To practice the most effective possible biological psychiatry, the psychopharmacologist also must learn to practice "six minute" psychotherapy.

SUMMARY: PSYCHODYNAMIC PSYCHOPHARMACOLOGY AND THE PATIENT-CENTERED TOOLKIT

The psychodynamic practice of psychiatry both can inform and improve the effectiveness of medication prescribing, and can include a limited but effective form of brief, supportive psychotherapy, as described by Michael and Enid Balint and by Mintz and Belnap. Technical recommendations to the psychodynamic psychiatric practitioner include the following: Avoid the mind-body split, understand the patient as a person, attend to the patient's ambivalence and resistance, cultivate the therapeutic alliance, be aware of the potential of countertherapeutic uses of medicine, and be aware of, manage, and use the feelings and reactions that arise in the clinical encounter both in patient and therapist.

REFERENCES

1. Laine C, Davidoff F. Patient-centered medicine. A professional evolution. JAMA 1996;275(2):152–6.
2. Sabshin M. Turning points in twentieth-century American psychiatry. Am J Psychiatry 1990;147(10):1267–74.
3. Kecmanovic D, Hadzi-Pavlovic D. Psychiatric journals as the mirror of the dominant psychiatric model. The Psychiatrist 2010;34(5):172–6. Available at: https://pdfs.semanticscholar.org/b672/81640fb744a8a7efcd4ef2edc5c8e3969ff9.pdf.
4. Mead N, Bower P. Patient-centredness: a conceptual framework and review of the empirical literature. Soc Sci Med 2000;51(7):1087–110.
5. Chong WW, Aslani P, Chen TF. Health care providers' perspectives of medication adherence in the treatment of depression: a qualitative study. Soc Psychiatry Psychiatr Epidemiol 2013;48(10):1657–66.
6. Insel T, Cuthbert B, Garvey M, et al. Research Domain Criteria (RDoC): toward a new classification framework for research on mental disorders. Am J Psychiatry 2010;167(7):748–51.
7. Star neuroscientist Tom Insel leaves the google-spawned verily for... a startup? WIRED. Available at: https://www.wired.com/2017/05/star-neuroscientist-tom-insel-leaves-google-spawned-verily-startup/. Accessed October 27, 2017.
8. Curtin SC, Warner M, Hedegaard H. Increase in suicide in the United States, 1999-2014. NCHS Data Brief 2016;(241):1–8.
9. Mintz D, Belnap B. A view from Riggs: treatment resistance and patient authority - III. What is psychodynamic psychopharmacology? An approach to pharmacologic treatment resistance. J Am Acad Psychoanal Dyn Psychiatry 2006;34(4):581–601.
10. Balint M. The crisis of medical practice. Am J Psychoanal 2002;62(1):7–15.
11. Balint M, Ball DH, Hare ML. Training medical students in patient-centered medicine. Compr Psychiatry 1969;10(4):249–58.
12. Balint E. The possibilities of patient-centered medicine. J R Coll Gen Pract 1969; 17(82):269–76.
13. Balint E. A study of the doctor-patient relationship using randomly selected cases. J Coll Gen Pract 1967;13(2):163–73.
14. Institute of Medicine (US) Committee on Quality of Health Care in America. Crossing the quality chasm: a new health system for the 21st century. Washington, DC: National Academies Press (US); 2001.

15. Dixon L, Lieberman J. Psychiatry embraces patient-centered care. Psychiatric News 2014;49(3):1.
16. Balint M. The doctor, his patient and the illness. London: Pitman Medical Publishing Co; 1964.
17. Balint M. The basic fault: therapeutic aspects of regression. London: Tavistock Publications; 1979.
18. Gabbard GO. Psychodynamic psychiatry in the "decade of the brain." Am J Psychiatry 1992;149(8):991–8.
19. Blagys MD, Hilsenroth MJ. Distinctive feature of short-term psychodynamic-interpersonal psychotherapy: a review of the comparative psychotherapy process literature. Clin Psychol Sci Pract 2000;7(2):167–88.
20. Abbass A, Luyten P, Steinert C, et al. Bias toward psychodynamic therapy: framing the problem and working toward a solution. J Psychiatr Pract 2017; 23(5):361–5.
21. Leichsenring F, Luyten P, Hilsenroth MJ, et al. Psychodynamic therapy meets evidence-based medicine: a systematic review using updated criteria. Lancet Psychiatry 2015;2(7):648–60.
22. Mintz DL, Flynn DF. How (not what) to prescribe: nonpharmacologic aspects of psychopharmacology. Psychiatr Clin North Am 2012;35(1):143–63.
23. Oestreicher C. A history of chaos theory. Dialogues Clin Neurosci 2007;9(3): 279–89. Available at: http://www.ncbi.nlm.nih.gov/pmc/articles/PMC3202497/.
24. Chalmers DJ. Facing up to the problem of consciousness. J Conscious Stud 1995;2(3):200–19.
25. Lueken U, Straube B, Konrad C, et al. Neural substrates of treatment response to cognitive-behavioral therapy in panic disorder with agoraphobia. Am J Psychiatry 2013;170:1345–55.
26. Karlsson H. Psychotherapy increases brain serotonin 5-HT1A receptors in patients with major depressive disorder. Psychol Med 2010;40:523–8.
27. Stahl SM. Psychotherapy as an epigenetic 'drug': psychiatric therapeutics target symptoms linked to malfunctioning brain circuits with psychotherapy as well as with drugs. J Clin Pharm Ther 2012;37(3):249–53.
28. Cross-Disorder Group of the Psychiatric Genomics Consortium, Lee SH, Ripke S, Neale BM, et al. Genetic relationship between five psychiatric disorders estimated from genome-wide SNPs. Nat Genet 2013;45(9):984–94.
29. Edwards VJ, Holden GW, Felitti VJ, et al. Relationship between multiple forms of childhood maltreatment and adult mental health in community respondents: results from the adverse childhood experiences study. Am J Psychiatry 2003; 160(8):1453–60.
30. Felitti VJ, Anda RF, Nordenberg D, et al. Relationship of childhood abuse and household dysfunction to many of the leading causes of death in adults: the adverse childhood experiences (ACE) study. Am J Prev Med 1998;14(4):245–58.
31. Kessler RC, McLaughlin KA, Green JG, et al. Childhood adversities and adult psychopathology in the WHO World Mental Health Surveys. Br J Psychiatry 2010;197(5):378–85.
32. Varese F, Smeets F, Drukker M, et al. Childhood adversities increase the risk of psychosis: a meta-analysis of patient-control, prospective- and cross-sectional cohort studies. Schizophr Bull 2012;38(4):661–71.
33. van Os J, McGuffin P. Can the social environment cause schizophrenia? Br J Psychiatry 2003;182:291–2.
34. Veling W, Susser E, van Os J, et al. Ethnic density of neighborhoods and incidence of psychotic disorders among immigrants. Am J Psychiatry 2008;165(1):66–73.

35. Selten J-P, Cantor-Graae E. Social defeat: risk factor for schizophrenia? Br J Psychiatry 2005;187(2):101–2.
36. Caspi A, Sugden K, Moffitt TE, et al. Influence of life stress on depression: moderation by a polymorphism in the 5-HTT gene. Science 2003;301(5631):386–9.
37. Caspi A, Hariri AR, Holmes A, et al. Genetic sensitivity to the environment: the case of the serotonin transporter gene and its implications for studying complex diseases and traits. Am J Psychiatry 2010;167(5):509–27.
38. Engel GL. The need for a new medical model: a challenge for biomedicine. Science 1977;196(4286):129–36.
39. Perry S, Cooper AM, Michels R. The psychodynamic formulation: its purpose, structure, and clinical application. Am J Psychiatry 1987;144(5):543–50.
40. Quilty LC, De Fruyt F, Rolland J-P, et al. Dimensional personality traits and treatment outcome in patients with major depressive disorder. J Affect Disord 2008; 108(3):241–50.
41. Davis C, Ralevski E, Kennedy SH, et al. The role of personality factors in the reporting of side effect complaints to moclobemide and placebo: a study of healthy male and female volunteers. J Clin Psychopharmacol 1995;15(5):347–52.
42. Kronström K, Salminen JK, Hietala J, et al. Does defense style or psychological mindedness predict treatment response in major depression? Depress Anxiety 2009;26(7):689–95.
43. Reynaert C, Janne P, Vause M, et al. Clinical trials of antidepressants: the hidden face: where locus of control appears to play a key role in depression outcome. Psychopharmacology (Berl) 1995;119(4):449–54.
44. Kirsch I, Moore TJ, Scoboria A, et al. The emperor's new drugs: an analysis of antidepressant medication data submitted to the U.S. Food and Drug Administration. Prevention and Treatment 2002;5:23.
45. de Craen AJ, Roos PJ, de Vries AL, et al. Effect of colour of drugs: systematic review of perceived effect of drugs and of their effectiveness. BMJ 1996; 313(7072):1624–6.
46. Waber RL, Shiv B, Carmon Z, et al. Commercial features of placebo and therapeutic efficacy. JAMA 2008;299(9):1016–7.
47. Kaptchuk TJ, Kelley JM, Conboy LA, et al. Components of placebo effect: randomised controlled trial in patients with irritable bowel syndrome. BMJ 2008; 336(7651):999–1003.
48. Hahn RA. The nocebo phenomenon: concept, evidence, and implications for public health. Prev Med 1997;26(5 Pt 1):607–11.
49. Mitsikostas DD, Mantonakis L, Chalarakis N. Nocebo in clinical trials for depression: a meta-analysis. Psychiatry Res 2014;215(1):82–6.
50. Barsky AJ. Nonpharmacologic aspects of medication. Arch Intern Med 1983; 143(8):1544–8.
51. Jensen KB, Kaptchuk TJ, Kirsch I, et al. Nonconscious activation of placebo and nocebo pain responses. Proc Natl Acad Sci U S A 2012;109(39):15959–64.
52. Mckay K, Imel Z, Wampold B. Psychiatrist effects in the psychopharmacological treatment of depression. J Affect Disord 2006;92:287–90.
53. Ankarberg P, Falkenström F. Treatment of depression with antidepressants is primarily a psychological treatment. Psychotherapy (Chic) 2008;45(3):329–39.
54. van Os TWDP, van den Brink RHS, Tiemens BG, et al. Communicative skills of general practitioners augment the effectiveness of guideline-based depression treatment. J Affect Disord 2005;84(1):43–51.
55. Zetzel ER. Current concepts of transference. Int J Psychoanal 1956;37:369–75.

56. Greenson RR. The working alliance and the transference neurosis. Psychoanal Q 1965;34:155–81.
57. Greenson RRW. The non-transference relationship in the psychoanalytic situation. Int J Psychoanal 1969;50:27–39.
58. Krupnick JL, Sotsky SM, Simmens S, et al. The role of the therapeutic alliance in psychotherapy and pharmacotherapy outcome: findings in the National Institute of Mental Health Treatment of Depression Collaborative Research Program. J Consult Clin Psychol 1996;64(3):532–9.
59. Sylvia LG, Hay A, Ostacher MJ, et al. Association between therapeutic alliance, care satisfaction, and pharmacological adherence in bipolar disorder. J Clin Psychopharmacol 2013;33(3):343–50.
60. Kaplan SH, Greenfield S, Ware JE. Assessing the effects of physician-patient interactions on the outcomes of chronic disease. Med Care 1989;27(3 Suppl): S110–27.
61. Woolley SB, Fredman L, Goethe JW, et al. Hospital patients' perceptions during treatment and early discontinuation of serotonin selective reuptake inhibitor antidepressants. J Clin Psychopharmacol 2010;30(6):716–9.
62. Gutheil TG. Drug therapy: alliance and compliance. Psychosomatics 1978;19(4): 219–25.
63. Aronson JK. Compliance, concordance, adherence. Br J Clin Pharmacol 2007; 63(4):383–4.
64. Sajatovic M, Ignacio RV, West JA, et al. Predictors of non-adherence among individuals with bipolar disorder receiving treatment in a community mental health clinic. Compr Psychiatry 2009;50(2):100–7.
65. Howes OD, McCutcheon R, Agid O, et al. Treatment-resistant schizophrenia: treatment response and resistance in psychosis (TRRIP) working group consensus guidelines on diagnosis and terminology. Am J Psychiatry 2016; 174(3):216–29.
66. Jamison KR, Gerner RH, Goodwin FK. Patient and physician attitudes toward lithium: relationship to compliance. Arch Gen Psychiatry 1979;36(8):866–9.
67. Moritz S, Hünsche A, Lincoln T. Nonadherence to antipsychotics: the role of positive attitudes towards positive symptoms. Eur Neuropsychopharmacol 2014;24: 1745–52.
68. Huhn M, Tardy M, Spineli LM, et al. Efficacy of pharmacotherapy and psychotherapy for adult psychiatric disorders: a systematic overview of meta-analyses. JAMA Psychiatry 2014;71(6):706–15.
69. Gabbard GO, Kay J. The fate of integrated treatment: whatever happened to the biopsychosocial psychiatrist? Am J Psychiatry 2001;158(12):1956–63.
70. Freud S. On Psychotherapy (1905 [1904]). In: Strachey J, Freud A, Richards A, et al, editors. The Standard edition of the complete psychological works of Sigmund Freud. London: Hogarth Press; 1966.
71. Wampold BE. How important are the common factors in psychotherapy? An update. World Psychiatr 2015;14(3):270–7.

Trauma-Focused Psychodynamic Psychotherapy

Fredric N. Busch, MD[a,b,c,*], Barbara L. Milrod, MD[a,b,c,d]

KEYWORDS

- Psychodynamic psychotherapy • Posttraumatic stress disorder
- Manualized psychotherapies • Intrapsychic conflict • Defense mechanisms
- Transference

KEY POINTS

- Despite the development of multiple approaches to posttraumatic stress disorder (PTSD), many patients do not respond or only partially respond to these interventions.
- The authors describe a psychodynamic psychotherapeutic approach to PTSD, derived from Panic-Focused Psychodynamic Psychotherapy, eXtended Range, which has demonstrated efficacy in treatment of panic disorder.
- This focused psychotherapy works to address disruptions in narrative coherence and affective dysregulation by exploring the psychological meanings of symptoms and their relation to traumatic events.
- The therapist works to identify intrapsychic conflicts, intense negative affects, and defense mechanisms related to PTSD symptoms in a psychodynamic formulation that provides a framework for treatment.
- The transference provides a forum for patients to address feelings of mistrust, difficulties with authority, fears of abuse, and angry and guilty feelings and fantasies.

INTRODUCTION

As per the *Diagnostic and Statistical Manual of Mental Disorders, Fifth Edition* (DSM-V),[1] posttraumatic stress disorder (PTSD) involves the development of a particular set of symptoms following exposure to traumatic events. The core features of

Dr B.L. Milrod's work was supported in part through a Fund in the New York Community; Trust established by DeWitt Wallace and a grant through the Weill Cornell Clinical; Translational Science Center Grant/Protocol Number: UL1 TR000457.
[a] 65 East 76th Street, Suite 1B, New York, NY 10021, USA; [b] Weill Cornell Medical College, 525 East 68th Street, New York, NY 10021, USA; [c] Columbia University Center for Psychoanalytic Training and Research, 1051 Riverside Drive, New York, NY 10032, USA; [d] The New York Psychoanalytic Institute, 247 East 82nd Street, New York, NY 10028, USA
* Corresponding author.
E-mail address: fnb80@aol.com

Psychiatr Clin N Am 41 (2018) 277–287
https://doi.org/10.1016/j.psc.2018.01.005

PTSD include distress from and avoidance of reminders of the triggering event(s), pervasive negative mood and thoughts, intrusive experiences related to trauma (eg, memories, dreams, flashbacks), insomnia, and hypervigilance. PTSD has a lifetime prevalence ranging from 1.3% to 12.2%.[2]

A variety of psychotherapeutic approaches and psychopharmacological treatments have been used for treatment of PTSD.[3] Various forms of cognitive behavioral therapy, which reviews and reexposes patients to traumatic events in a controlled setting, along with addressing associated avoidance and cognitive distortions, are in the class of psychological therapies for PTSD that have the most empirical support.[4] Other psychotherapeutic approaches with some evidence base include interpersonal therapy, which targets interpersonal conflicts and role transitions,[5] and stair narrative therapy,[6] which focuses on skills training in affect management and interpersonal difficulties, along with development of a narrative to identify meaning in traumatic experiences. A variety of innovative or alternative treatments also have been used, including eye movement desensitization reflex, transcranial magnetic stimulation, and neurofeedback.[3] However, response without remission and nonresponse rates remain high across treatments[4] and psychodynamic psychotherapy has undergone little systematic study.

Our research group has developed and is testing a psychodynamic psychotherapeutic approach targeting PTSD: trauma-focused psychodynamic psychotherapy (TFPP). This treatment was derived from Panic-Focused Psychodynamic Psychotherapy—eXtended Range (PFPP-XR),[7] the first psychodynamically based psychotherapy to have demonstrated efficacy as a sole treatment for a DSM-IV anxiety disorder, specifically panic disorder with or without agoraphobia, in 3 randomized controlled trials.[8,9] The PFPP-XR treatment manual discusses a psychodynamic formulation and specific approaches to PTSD, and several research studies using PFPP-XR have included patients with PTSD.[8–10] PFPP-XR has been studied as a 24-session, 12-week treatment; the appropriate length of TFPP is currently being evaluated. We describe the psychodynamic formulation and basic treatment approaches for PTSD (TFPP) based on this clinical and research experience.

CORE PSYCHODYNAMIC FACTORS IN POSTTRAUMATIC STRESS DISORDER

The Impact of Trauma on Mind and Self

Neurophysiological and psychological influences that occur during traumatic experiences disrupt memory consolidation and trigger powerful emotions. This impact has the following consequences:

- Memory disruptions can undermine the individual's sense of self as continuous and predictable.
- Moments of terrifying clarity, which sometimes accompany flashbacks, alternate with hazy impressions about the traumatic events, impeding a coherent narrative of the trauma and its emotional impact.
- Affective dysregulation is common, with a patient's emotions emerging unpredictably and with a sense of perplexing discontinuity.

Understanding and articulating these central elements of the traumatic experience are crucial to working psychodynamically to help PTSD patients develop a more coherent narrative regarding their traumatic experiences. As discussed in this article, these efforts are important in developing self-understanding of emotions, thoughts, and internal conflicts that contribute to persistent symptoms, as well as in developing a more coherent sense of self after trauma.

Repetition

A core aspect of the psychoanalytic understanding of PTSD is the idea that traumatic experiences can be unconsciously repeated.[11,12] What has been overwhelming and remains psychically unintegrated may be repeated in the following ways:

- The patient may experience an objectively dissimilar set of circumstances as a recurrence of the trauma, or
- The patient may unconsciously enter into and at times even provoke experiences reminiscent of the trauma. Such repetitions often represent unconscious efforts to master or control traumatic experiences during which individuals felt powerless.

Intrapsychic Conflict

Discomfort about contradictory, concurrent, and often mixed wishes and fantasies and internalized prohibitions about them are referred to as "intrapsychic conflict," a core psychodynamic principle regarding the functioning of the mind. Intrapsychic conflicts are considered to play a central role in symptom formation and the triggering of defenses that unconsciously attempt to avert the conscious emergence of wishes or impulses about which there are mixed feelings. For example, key areas of psychodynamic conflict in anxiety disorders include conflicted feelings about autonomy, separation from close, ambivalently held attachment figures, difficulty tolerating anger, and guilty self-punishment.[7] Patients with panic disorder often struggle with rageful feelings and fantasies toward an important attachment figure, but fear their anger could lead to a potential disruption of this essential relationship. The potential emergence of these wishes into consciousness triggers significant anxiety and panic.

Identifying and understanding intrapsychic conflicts are pivotal components of TFPP. Prominent examples of conflicts in PTSD include the following:

- Rageful reactions to the trauma can trigger exaggerated guilt about wishes to harm others.
- Patients struggle with wishes to be closer to others, but are terrified that others will reject or abuse them, repeating their traumatic experiences.

Traumatic experiences trigger complex emotions and fantasies that are fertile ground for the development of intrapsychic conflict. Feelings of intense rage at those who have perpetrated harm or allowed harm to happen can conflict with fears of loss and disrupted attachments increased by a mistrust of others. Conflicted feelings of anger, sadness, and abandonment often emerge toward an important attachment figure who is an aggressor. In examining these complex feelings and fantasies, TFPP provides a means of identifying and untangling sources of conflict to aid patients in developing a better understanding of their struggles and more adaptive internal representations.

Dissociation and Other Defenses

Trauma survivors defend themselves against the full implications of their traumatic experiences, associated conflicted fantasies, and often unbearable feelings of pain, humiliation, rage, helplessness, and severe anxiety that accompany them, via various unconscious defensive maneuvers. Although any defense mechanism may serve this function, certain defenses are more predominant in PTSD, including *dissociation, repression, a counterphobic stance, and identification with the aggressor*. In their various forms, these defense mechanisms represent different ways of avoiding painful feelings and fantasies, often linked to traumatic experiences. Identifying specific defenses aids the therapist in addressing and clarifying them with the patient, allowing greater access to underlying painful and frightening memories, feelings, and fantasies.

Dissociation
Dissociation represents a mechanism by which patients feel disconnected from others, reality, or their own emotional states. For example, an individual may speak of a traumatic event while consciously experiencing an absence of emotion, or numbness. Dissociative states, such as pervasive numbing, are an unconscious means of avoiding the pain associated with the trauma. Dissociative states can alternate with intense affects, including anxiety, triggered by reminders of the horror experienced, with the reemergence of painful aspects of the trauma (intrusive memories, intense emotions, and visceral flashbacks). Individuals may also attempt to defend against the reemergence of the memory or its reminders through avoidance, including certain people or activities felt to be associated with the trauma. In approaching dissociation, the therapist works to link emotions, fantasies, and memories that are disconnected from each other, and tracks the sense of dissociation in terms of when and how it occurs, and its associated fantasies.

Repression
Repression represents an unconscious mechanism through which feelings, fantasies, and memories that create pain and anxiety are kept from conscious awareness. For example, patients may repress wishes to be taken care of, as they do not want to be vulnerable to others' harming them. In dealing with repression, the therapist works to bring to consciousness affects and fantasies that are out of awareness.

Counterphobic stance
Some survivors maintain a *counterphobic stance* that serves to deny the extent of the impact of the trauma. For example, a woman sexually abused as a child might, out of her awareness, become promiscuous, to both ragefully punish men and also to deny the experience of her own helplessness and vulnerability to harm. This counterphobic behavior may result in the patient's repeatedly putting herself in harm's way, making her vulnerable to further trauma. In these instances, the therapist helps the patient identify how these behaviors and attitudes attempt to avert the patient's fears, while actually creating greater risks.

Identification with the aggressor
In using the defense mechanism of *identification with the aggressor*, patients connect their own image of themselves with that of an aggressive individual, particularly someone who has had power over them in the past. In this way, individuals can identify with perpetrators of the trauma, with compelling fantasies/wishes of being powerful and invulnerable, and hurting others as they themselves were hurt. These fantasies can trigger significant guilt and are often kept out of awareness.

Guilt and Shame

In PTSD, patients' symptoms are often connected to conscious or unconscious guilt and shame about some aspect of the traumatic experience itself or their role in it, and associated conflicted feelings and fantasies, for which they feel compelled to punish themselves:

- Traumatized individuals may have internalized the sense of dehumanization and disgust with which a tormentor, rapist, or assailant treated them, and may consciously experience this as a part of themselves for which they deserve to be punished or humiliated.

- "Survivor guilt" can arise from conflicts about having survived a trauma when others died or were more severely injured.
- As noted previously, the effort to avoid a sense of helplessness with fantasies of damaging others linked to identification with the aggressor can trigger intense guilt and self-disgust.

BEGINNING THE TREATMENT: ENGAGING THE PATIENT IN A PSYCHOLOGICALLY BASED THERAPY

Some patients readily engage in the psychotherapeutic process, making an effort to understand the psychological origins of their PTSD symptoms. Others show little interest, due to character style, lack of familiarity with unconscious mental life, inability to see the relevance of psychological issues to their symptoms, or defensive denial. The therapist can often rapidly engage patients' interest and curiosity by demonstrating how symptoms may be related to patients' traumatic histories and current and past mode of conducting themselves. The therapist can connect the anxiety and its associated fantasies with ongoing emotional concerns that the patient has had since the traumatic event or even throughout his or her life.

Developing the patient's capacity for psychological-mindedness is an important part of psychodynamic psychotherapeutic work. The therapist actively provides useful examples of psychological factors that emerge in the patient's symptoms. Patients can generally use this material, and usually can elaborate on the formulations presented by the therapist, adding details and altering the formulation to apply to their situation more exactly. This is part of the process of developing the capacity to *reflect on* one's symptoms, a key element of dynamic therapy. TFPP also uses core techniques of psychodynamic psychotherapy, including clarification, confrontation, and interpretation.

Attending to Mistrust, Disruptions in Narrative Coherence, Shame, and Terror

In the initial sessions of TFPP, the therapist embarks on an effort with patients to understand the impact of recent and past traumas on their lives, thereby relieving symptoms. Certain core features of PTSD can complicate this task, including disruptions of patients' (1) basic sense of trust, and (2) narrative coherence. In addition, traumatized patients often feel deeply ashamed and guilt-ridden, repeatedly questioning themselves about whether they could have done something to prevent the traumatic event or whether something they did contributed to the event. They are often enraged at others not affected by trauma, or those who cannot understand their experience in some way. They may wish to avoid discussing it and have frequently unconsciously disconnected from aspects of the most troublesome and painful feelings or memories. At the same time, they often live in conscious and unconscious terror that the trauma could recur at any time, and they may have extreme difficulty ever feeling safe. They may retreat from others in an effort to protect themselves, but then feel isolated. Their terror, sense of being constantly under threat, isolation, dissociation, and consequent hopelessness can complicate the work and makes it important for the therapist to be particularly sensitive to these vulnerabilities.

Despite these problems, a therapist's efforts to relieve anxiety and distrust can address concerns that patients may have kept to themselves, believing that others could not tolerate their feelings or help to relieve them. The therapist works on building a safe enough therapeutic relationship for the patient to address traumatic experiences, gradually helping them to tolerate their impact and meaning. It is essential that the therapist not force patients to describe feelings or situations that they are reluctant to address, as this may repeat the traumatic encounter, in which the therapist can be seen as the aggressor. The therapist attempts to address feelings that have been "frozen" or static, which have greatly affected the patient's mental life. It may be useful to acknowledge that the patient's reactions and feelings are an understandable response to the traumatic event(s).

Exploration of Traumatic Events and Associated Symptoms

In TFPP, symptoms serve as a lens through which to identify the patient's symptoms, conflicts, and defenses and to understand their genesis. The therapist obtains information about symptoms and the associated context and feelings, and considers how these elements may carry emotional links to the trauma. As soon as is tactfully feasible, the therapist explores what the patient can relate about the traumatic event(s), including details of the event(s) and emotional reactions to them. The patient will often not be comfortable or able to provide a complete story. The therapist mentally, and sometimes verbally to the patient, notes gaps, confusions, and inconsistencies in the presentation of events, as these may indicate painful or conflicted aspects that have triggered dissociation or self-loathing. The therapist may gently begin to explore these gaps, but must remain alert that this foray may feel traumatic to the patient, perhaps causing an adverse emotional reaction. It is important to explore what the patient believes are the impacts of the traumatic event(s) at the time they occurred, subsequently, and in current life, as well as his or her ongoing fantasies about the meaning of the trauma.

Exploration of Meaning of Symptoms

In the initial phase, the therapist explores the underlying psychological antecedents (that is, early events and circumstances that might explain the patient's outlook) and (unconscious) emotional meanings of various symptoms. The therapist seeks to identify the meanings of somatic symptoms, including memories of bodily experiences associated with the trauma and may link certain sensations to aspects of the traumatic situation, such as time of day, lighting, location, noises, music, and smells. These sensory cues can be extremely powerful and can make the patient feel vividly and suddenly back in the traumatic situation. The therapist explores the functions of dissociative numbing, which can be an unconscious means of disconnecting from the pain of the trauma, while at the same time keeping it in mind, as numbing can serve as a reminder of the state the trauma induced. The therapist seeks to identify the many ways, often involving unwitting reenactments of traumatic relationships, in which nightmares, flashbacks, and feeling states continue to intrude into consciousness and get replayed. The therapist explores how symptoms of reexperiencing may unconsciously keep the trauma in one's mind without consciously focusing on or thinking about it. Another possible meaning is that these reexperiences signify or recreate important aspects of relationships, such as with a controlling and punitive parent, or an abuser in the context of trauma. These are among many potential compelling unconscious mechanisms that can decrease in intensity when they are openly explored.

Exploration of Past Traumas

People who already feel personally insecure and unsafe and suffer from separation anxiety or insecure attachments are more vulnerable to PTSD.[13] It is therefore important to identify whether patients have had past traumatic experiences or insecure formative attachment relationships, and the nature of their subsequent impact. Determining these undercurrents is not necessarily a straightforward endeavor, as patients with PTSD commonly have difficulty tolerating/accepting the degree of their disappointment and rage at close attachment figures who may have been responsible for childhood trauma. The therapist should explore patients' developmental history for adverse events, such as severe family conflict and physical or sexual abuse. Family management of emotions, including anger, shame, and anxiety is also vital information, as this history reveals much about patients' state of mind when confronted with trauma. Probes include the following:

- How do you feel about these events in your past?
- Are you enraged, guilty, self-blaming, ashamed?
- Are you aware that numbness may be a way of avoiding painful "hot button" aspects of the trauma?
- How do these events affect your sense of yourself and expectations of others?
- How has trauma affected your sense of trust?

The therapist should help the patient to identify links from the past to more recent experiences.

Reexperiencing of Traumas

Therapists using TFPP work to identify and explore symptoms that represent reexperiencing of the trauma. These can include nightmares, flashbacks, or feeling as if the trauma is recurring in the present. The therapist identifies that there are reasons why patients continue to relive these particular aspects of the trauma, and that understanding why they occur when they do as well as their underlying emotional antecedents can provide inroads to recognizing a deeper psychological basis for these symptoms. Contributors to persistent reexperiencing may include unaddressed guilt, rage, or disruptions in identity or sense of cohesion. This reliving can also represent an unconscious attempt to undo loss and magically repair fractured relationships.

Repetition of the Trauma

It is valuable for patients to grow aware that they may unconsciously repeat aspects of the trauma or perceive benign situations as traumatic. Patients typically find this counterintuitive, as they often feel convinced that they try everything possible to avoid repeating the traumatic experience. However, several factors may contribute to such a repetition, including averting intolerable feelings of helplessness surrounding the trauma by "getting it right" or seeking control. Additionally, patients may repeat the trauma as an unconscious self-punishment for an aspect of themselves/their fantasies that they feel guilty about, such as survivor guilt or a wish to harm and abuse as they were harmed. The therapist helps patients to identify when they perceive benign situations as traumatic, and how trauma influences their misperception.

Exploration of Guilt and a Sense of "Badness"

Guilt often accompanies interpersonal trauma, and it is important to explore contributors to this guilt with the patient to help relieve it. These sources can include survivor guilt, in which patients feel guilty that they survived while others did not. Patients may be overwhelmed with guilt about having protected themselves or others violently. They may believe that they could have done something to prevent the traumatic event(s), obsessively reviewing the circumstances of the event(s) with a focus on how they might have intervened in some way. The therapist works with the patient to identify how there is a sense of overresponsibility, with a fantasy that the patient could have controlled what happened, undoing helpless intolerable feelings. Another source of significant guilt is patients' rage, including at those who perpetrated or could have prevented the trauma or those unaffected by the trauma. They may feel guilty about wishes or fantasies to harm others as they were harmed, as in identifying with the aggressor. Patients may unconsciously arrange to punish themselves or others regarding some aspect of the trauma about which they feel guilty and have not permitted themselves to consider or address (eg, feeling guilty that they survived, being flooded with unacceptably aggressive fantasies).

In the context of severe trauma, patients often view themselves as "bad," triggered by guilt and conflicted anger at others directed toward the self. Patients may also view themselves negatively to protect against intolerably painful perceptions of others as cruel, damaging, and terrorizing. This sense of personal badness may also paradoxically allow fantasies of greater control: they see themselves as less helpless if they themselves are to blame, rather than uncontrollable others.

Identification with the Aggressor

Patients are understandably enraged after experiencing trauma, including against those who perpetrated the trauma or those who put them in harm's way. However, people with PTSD often have difficulty identifying, acknowledging, or expressing their anger appropriately. This inability to access rage can be due to guilt or anxiety that their rage may become out of control or damage others. In other instances, rage may be unmanageable, with seemingly out-of-control, dissociated explosive outbursts, and additional interventions may be required, such as medication. Individuals frequently identify with those who have harmed them, as they connect emotionally with the power and control they ascribe to the abuser. Patients may find themselves, disturbingly, fantasizing about harming others as they were harmed. For example, those who have been bullied may have a wish to bully others or may engage in such bullying. However, the patient may struggle with tremendous guilt about fantasies of revenge. It is important to explore with patients the nature of their rage, revenge fantasies, or wishes to harm others. Many of these fantasies directly trigger anxiety, panic, and guilt. The therapist's role in these instances includes helping patients to tolerate their rage, permitting them to articulate fantasies openly, pointing out that these fantasies make sense in the context of the trauma and are not dangerous in and of themselves. To the extent that patients may be acting out these behaviors, therapists will need to help them understand the origins of these impulses while finding better ways of coping with their anger. This requires that therapists themselves tolerate the rage that arises in the sessions.[14]

THE MIDDLE PHASE OF TREATMENT: IDENTIFYING AND ELABORATING CORE DYNAMICS

Core components of the middle phase of TFPP include the development of a psychodynamic formulation centered on the patient's PTSD, an increased understanding of the dynamics through exploration and interpretation of the transference, and working through.

Psychodynamic Formulation

Within the first few sessions, therapists should provide a preliminary psychodynamic formulation regarding the impact of the trauma on the patient's fears, anxiety, and sense of personal coherence. In addition to identifying meanings of symptoms and relevant conflicts and defenses, the formulation in TFPP is particularly important for structuring a more coherent narrative for the patient. Typical dynamics include conflicts over rage and identification with the aggressor, with accompanying feelings of guilt and shame; helplessness and vulnerability and a fear that others cannot be trusted; a persistent sense of disruption and incoherence, including a dissociative tendency with diminished access to relevant emotional states; and a dangerous unconscious pull toward repetition. The formulation will be added to and adjusted throughout the middle phase of the treatment (and often into the termination phase), developing a framework for increased insight and integration.

Exploration of the Transference

Each of the various feelings, conflicts, and defenses that arise in therapy can emerge in relation to feelings and fantasies about the therapist, referred to as the transference. Although transference interpretations are typically used after several sessions, they may be used early when problems in the therapeutic relationship threaten to disrupt the treatment, including when the patient becomes frightened or wary about talking or otherwise expresses distrust of the therapist. Patients with PTSD typically have had multiple problematic experiences in relation to authority and their sense of security and safety in the world. Given these issues, it is important to monitor and address whether indeed patients view the therapist as a helper. It is likely that patients will experience or develop some wariness about their therapist, as this frequently becomes a dominant mode for these patients in most if not all relationships subsequent to the traumatic event(s). The transference provides an important opportunity to explore this wariness with the patient.

Additionally, patients will almost certainly react with ambivalence to the therapist's efforts to address the painful experience of the trauma as well as difficult feelings surrounding the event. Patients may become frustrated or disconnect from the therapist's efforts. If this happens, it is important to point this out to the patient, ask the patient what his or her experience of these conversations is, and attempt to pinpoint why the patient feels disengaged when he or she does. The therapist not only needs tact in encouraging the patient to explore the trauma, but also to acknowledge the difficulties in addressing painful feelings and memories.

Patients may view the therapist as an aggressor or abuser, potentially retraumatizing them, or may become enraged or have fantasies of harming the therapist as revenge or as part of identification with the aggressor. Articulating and exploring anger and whether these patients feel enraged or threatened is crucial. These reactions present an opportunity to learn more about the patient's internal struggles. Patients also may have a sense of themselves as toxic and poisonous to the therapist. Guilt may arise in conjunction with these feelings and can provide additional clues about areas of difficulty arising from the trauma.

Countertransference with Patients with Posttraumatic Stress Disorder

Patients with PTSD present particular countertransference difficulties. Therapists may find the pain of the patient's traumatic experiences particularly difficult to tolerate. Therapists should be alert to their own distress and the potential to inadvertently steer the patient away from difficult topics, colluding with patient avoidance, and aggravating the patient's sense of his or her own toxicity. Therapists also may identify with the patient's sense of helplessness and sometimes feel helpless themselves. At these points, it is important for them to recall that talking with the patient about his or her pain and trying to articulate its fluctuations (eg, what makes it better and worse) aids in developing a road map for the relief of symptoms. Just having someone with whom to share suffering who can tolerate blasts of negative affect[14] usually provides both relief of painful feelings and hope for change. Patients' inner feelings of fragmentation can sometimes create discomfort for therapists, perhaps pressing them to create a narrative more rapidly than is reasonable, as aspects of the trauma typically emerge slowly as trust is gradually built, over time. Therapists also need to learn to tolerate the patients viewing them as abusers, while helping to address these misperceptions.

Working Through

Working through is a gradual process in which the patient's acquired knowledge of conflicts and psychic functioning are steadily applied to increase his or her understanding of how these conflicts affect various areas of the patient's life and symptoms. This phase helps to reduce the patient's vulnerability to PTSD symptoms, as various ramifications of central conflicts and contributing factors to this vulnerability are explored. In the psychotherapeutic situation, the process is marked by repeating similar interpretations as they apply to different manifestations of the same intrapsychic phenomenon. The patient begins to appreciate how pervasively this particular set of dynamics has affected him or her. The patient typically demonstrates improved functioning in work and relationships as the patient becomes more conscious of his or her conflicts and their impact.

Therapists must be aware that patients rarely change in response to a single interpretation, no matter how central; a gradual accretion of clarifications and interpretations is usually necessary. In addition, interpretations may be rephrased and modified by the patient, who brings them into closer approximation to his or her own experience.

Because patients with anxiety and PTSD have inherent difficulty connecting their often-overwhelming feelings with intellectually understandable ideas, the working-through process is essential in making connections between different aspects of the patient's intrapsychic experience and life and developing a coherent self-narrative. The therapist continues to work with the patient on feelings of alienation, incoherence, dissociation, badness, guilt, mistrust, and feeling endangered, while further addressing conflicts surrounding anger and identification with the aggressor. Evidence of working through includes the patient's increasing awareness of the nature of symptom triggers, and a new ability to effectively manage the challenges and emotions brought up in these situations.

Working through occurs outside of therapeutic sessions as well, as patients ponder what has been said in treatment and recognize how it applies to their lives. As they develop a greater sense of cohesion and less mistrust in relationships, they often allow themselves to become closer to others. Better resolutions of old conflicts enable patients to take new chances that may have felt too risky to contemplate previously. Ideally, new ways of relating to others permit the patient to realize his or her desires to love and connect more with others, and to feel greater satisfaction and pleasure in all aspects of life.

TERMINATION

Ending the treatment and the patient's emotional response to this should be addressed as it arises throughout the therapy because of the patient's difficulties with past separations and losses. During termination, the patient will likely be responding to the impending loss of the therapist and feeling anger toward him or her as well as sadness. Distrust may reemerge. If the treatment has successfully engaged the patient, he or she will learn to cope with ending the relationship with someone who has provided relief from pain, who has paid careful attention, and who has enabled the patient to discuss difficult topics and feelings. A positive outcome includes the capacity to better address these struggles with others in the patient's life. Angry or anxious reactions about the relationship ending should be calmly explored from early stages of the treatment, and linked, where possible, to other disruptions in trust and sense of self-cohesion. Termination provides additional opportunities to identify painful and conflicted feelings and fantasies in the transference and when addressed openly in therapy, can help the patient to feel safer and more tolerant of these feelings. In addition, patients can become more aware of the ongoing impact of the trauma and take measures increasingly to think and behave in ways that promote greater self-esteem and better relationships. They can mourn the sense that the impact of the trauma might never entirely resolve, while also seeing that they can nonetheless live much more fulfilling lives with greater feelings of deepening connection.

REFERENCES

1. American Psychiatric Association. Diagnostic and statistical manual of mental disorders. 5th edition. Arlington (VA): American Psychiatric Press; 2013.
2. Karam EG, Friedman MJ, Hill ED, et al. Cumulative traumas and risk thresholds: 12-month PTSD in the World Mental Health (WMH) surveys. Depress Anxiety 2014;31:130–42.
3. Shalev A, Liberzon I, Marmar C. Post-traumatic stress disorder. N Engl J Med 2017;376:2459–69.
4. Steenkamp MM, Litz BT, Hoge CW, et al. Psychotherapy for military related PTSD: a review of randomized clinical trials. JAMA 2015;314:489–500.
5. Markowitz JC, Petkova E, Neria Y, et al. Is exposure necessary? A randomized clinical trial of interpersonal psychotherapy for PTSD. Am J Psychiatry 2015; 172:430–40.
6. Cloitre M, Stovall-McClough KC, Nooner K, et al. Treatment for PTSD related to childhood abuse: a randomized controlled trial. Am J Psychiatry 2010;167: 915–24.
7. Busch FN, Milrod BL, Singer M, et al. Panic-focused psychodynamic psychotherapy, eXtended range. New York: Routledge; 2012.
8. Milrod B, Leon AC, Busch FN, et al. A randomized controlled clinical trial of psychoanalytic psychotherapy for panic disorder. Am J Psychiatry 2007;164:265–72.
9. Milrod B, Chambless DL, Gallop R, et al. Psychotherapies for panic disorder: a tale of two sites. J Clin Psychiatry 2016;77:927–35.
10. Milrod B, Shapiro S, Gross C, et al. Does manualized psychodynamic psychotherapy have an impact on youth anxiety disorders? Am J Psychother 2013;67: 359–66.
11. Corradi RB. The repetition compulsion in psychodynamic psychotherapy. J Am Acad Psychoanal Dyn Psychiatry 2009;37:477–500.
12. Freud S. Beyond the pleasure principle. In: Strachey J, editor. The standard edition of the complete psychological works of Sigmund Freud, vol. 18. London: Hogarth Press; 1920. p. 1–64.
13. Silove D, Alonso J, Bromet E, et al. Psychotherapy for military related PTSD: a review of randomized clinical trials. JAMA 2015;314:489–500.
14. Markowitz JC, Milrod B. The importance of responding to negative affect in psychotherapies. Am J Psychiatry 2011;168:124–8.

Advocacy for Psychodynamic Psychotherapy

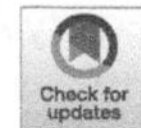

Challenges and Benefits

Katherine G. Kennedy, MD*

KEYWORDS

• Advocacy • Psychodynamic psychotherapy • Psychodynamic therapy • Challenges • Advocates

KEY POINTS

- Psychodynamic psychotherapy, also called psychodynamic therapy (PDT), is an effective and cost-effective mental health treatment.
- An array of factors, such as stigma, managed care reimbursement practices, and a bias toward pharmacotherapy, create barriers for patients to access PDT.
- To improve access to PDT, psychiatrists have a responsibility to advocate for changes in the current and future financial, regulatory, and attitudinal systems.
- Psychiatrists have not been trained in advocacy skills and face additional challenges to advocacy.
- Requisite advocacy skills and an approach to advocacy for PDT are described.

The American mental health care delivery system is undergoing a foundational transformation. The decisions made in the next few years will affect the way health care is organized and delivered for the next generation. Psychodynamic psychotherapy, also called psychodynamic therapy (PDT), is an effective mental health treatment that is currently under siege on several fronts. It is at risk of being effectively excluded from the future of American health care. Psychiatrists need to advocate for a future mental health care delivery system that ensures their patients have access to PDT and other quality mental health treatments.

Psychiatrists who practice PDT face increasing barriers. They must frequently allocate valuable patient time to preauthorization requests and other utilization review tasks. These chores detract from seeing patients and other professional responsibilities. Adding to this burden, managed care organizations routinely deny treatment, often at rates that defy the promise of parity created by the 2008 Mental Health Parity and Addiction

Disclosure Statement: No disclosures.
Department of Psychiatry, Yale Medical School, New Haven, CT, USA
* 66 Trumbull Street, New Haven, CT 06510.
E-mail address: katherine.kennedy@yale.edu

Psychiatr Clin N Am 41 (2018) 289–303
https://doi.org/10.1016/j.psc.2018.01.002
0193-953X/18/

Equity Act. As a preemptive move, some psychiatrists choose not to accept insurance. However, this creates financial barriers for many patients and does not address the underlying problem: the current PDT reimbursement system favors managed care organizations, puts the onus on psychiatrists, and punishes patients.

There are additional barriers to the practice of PDT: inadequate state insurance laws and regulations; lack of enforcement of current state and federal parity and insurance laws[1]; health care systems' exclusion of PDT from treatment options; public misperceptions about the benefits, efficacy, and cost of PDT; research bias against PDT[2]; the stigma against PDT by other physicians and non-PDT psychiatrists[3]; the pharmacology industry's substantial financial support for medication-only interventions; and inconsistent PDT training in psychiatric residency programs.

Psychiatrists need to advocate for systemic changes (financial, regulatory, and attitudinal) that facilitate their ability to practice PDT, improve patients' access to PDT, and eliminate unreasonable barriers to PDT. However, calls for vigorous advocacy for PDT[4] have gone largely unheeded. Psychiatrists may feel reluctant or unprepared to advocate. This article examines the challenges that prospective psychiatrist-advocates face and offers suggestions for an approach to advocacy for PDT. Psychiatrists need to advocate for PDT before the opportunity is gone.

THE BENEFITS OF PSYCHODYNAMIC THERAPY

PDT has a strong evidence base as an effective treatment.[5] A meta-analysis by Leichsenring and colleagues[6] demonstrated that PDT is highly effective in treating a range of psychiatric disorders with robust effect sizes that far surpass the effect sizes associated with many medication trials.[7] A 2017 meta-analysis by Steinert and colleagues[8] found that PDT is as efficacious as cognitive behavioral therapy, which has a well-established evidence base for efficacy. Also, a meta-analysis by Huhn and colleagues[9] found PDT to be as effective as pharmacotherapy. With many cohorts of patients, a combined medical and PDT approach for certain disorders has been shown to be more effective[10] and less complicated[11] than split treatment. In addition, when PDT is added to pharmacotherapy, the response rate for patients increases.[12]

PDT can lead to enduring psychological improvement, even after treatment has ended.[13] Furthermore, PDT has proven to be cost-effective for many psychiatric disorders, especially chronic complex disorders.[14,15] PDT has no medication-related side effects and has lower rates of dropout than medication alone.[5] Few adverse effects for PDT have been identified, although more research is needed in this area.[16]

PDT skills are foundational to the practice of psychiatry, such that the Accreditation Council for Graduate Medical Education requires psychiatry residency training programs to include PDT within their core competencies.[17] Although psychiatrists may ultimately specialize in other aspects of psychiatry, learning PDT skills is considered essential. As a result, psychiatrists receive the most intensive medical training and PDT education compared with all other providers, including pediatricians, internists, family practitioners, Advanced Practice Registered Nurses, and psychologists with prescribing privileges.

THE NEGATIVE PUBLIC PERCEPTION OF PSYCHIATRISTS

A recent online comment to an editorial read, "Psychiatry as a profession has been incredibly dishonest and manipulative, not to mention dogmatic and defensive when legitimate critiques are raised...When psychiatrists stop being arrogant know-it-alls who aren't really interested in either scientific data or their own patient's reactions to their vaunted 'treatments,' then maybe the well-deserved 'stigma' toward psychiatry might begin to abate."[18]

Diatribes against psychiatry abound in the blogosphere. But Internet trolls are only the latest in the line of those who ridicule psychiatry and psychiatrists. Cartoons of old, bearded men sitting beside couches with notepads in their hands populate *The New Yorker* and operate as universally recognized signifiers for all forms of therapy. The general public's perceptions have also been colored by books and movies such as *One Flew Over the Cuckoo's Nest*, in which psychiatrists shackle patients and medicate them against their will. When not viewed as authoritarian and dehumanizing, psychiatrists are condemned as passive, silent, eggheads who can read minds yet withhold helpful advice. Or they may be likened to Lucy, the lazy and self-serving *Peanuts* cartoon character who extorts money for wasteful talk therapy.

Moreover, these distorted perceptions are not confined to the general public.[19] A 2015 study by Stuart and colleagues[3] demonstrated that the "vast majority" of nonpsychiatric medical school teaching faculty, who are also academic medical doctors, regard psychiatrists as "unethical, exploitative, or mentally deranged."

A 2016 Gallup Poll[20] conducted to gauge the general public's perceptions of honesty and ethics in a variety of professions found that only 38% ranked psychiatrists as very high or high in these categories, in contrast to medical doctors, who received a 65% ranking of very high or high. Psychiatrists received the same ranking as chiropractors, although they did rank higher than business executives (at 17%) and Health Maintenance Organization managers (at 12%). A curious feature of the poll was that psychiatrists were the only medical professionals extracted from the category of medical doctors. The pollsters did not explain their rationale for the distinction; however, it suggests that they share the public's confusion[21] about the difference between psychiatrists and other mental health professionals, ignoring (or unaware of) the medical training of psychiatrists.

THE NEGATIVE OPTICS OF PSYCHODYNAMIC THERAPY

These negative optics extend to PDT, which has been maligned, distorted, and discounted as a valid treatment.[3] Even psychiatrists sometimes overlook PDT as an effective treatment tool. Multiple studies of so-called treatment-resistant disorders fail to offer psychotherapy as an intervention after traditional first-line medication trials fail. Instead, they suggest the use of off-label prescriptions or other drug interventions, despite the multiple randomized controlled studies that have demonstrated the efficacy of PDT[5–8]; and they overlook the benefits when PDT is added to medication.

About 30 years ago, a confluence of processes helped push the concept of PDT as a valid treatment out of consciousness (pun fully intended). These included:

- In the 1980 edition of the *Diagnostic and Statistical Manual of Mental Disorders*, 3rd edition (DSM-III), psychodynamic theory was eliminated from diagnostic categories and psychiatric diagnosis was reduced to a checklist of symptoms. DSM-III gave patients a psychiatric diagnosis when they demonstrated enough symptoms across certain categories, without regard to personal narrative. Absent psychodynamic theory, DSM-III essentially sidelined PDT from mental health treatments, while enabling the pharmaceutical industry to redefine mental health treatment as symptom-targeted drug therapy.
- In the 1980s, several psychoanalytic cases came to light in which antipsychotic and antidepressant medications were not offered to patients who might have benefitted; this seemed to reflect antipathy by many psychoanalysts toward adding medication to psychotherapy.
- Several new, effective psychotropic medications were identified (tricyclic antidepressants, selective serotonin reuptake inhibitors, clozapine), which spurred greater research and excitement about the promise of biological treatments.

- In 1989, Congress passed a resolution, affirmed by President George H.W. Bush's proclamation and supported by the National Institute of Mental Health that the 1990s would be the Decade of the Brain; this further propelled research into biological treatments and away from psychotherapy research.
- In 1990, *JAMA* published its first article of evidence-based medicine launching a movement for empirically based treatments.[22] Approaches such as PDT, which at that time had a limited evidence base, were correspondingly discredited.
- In the early 1990s, managed care organizations introduced more stringent utilization review processes, using more restrictive guidelines that were not consistent with best medical practices and often developed by nonclinicians to lower costs rather than improve patient health; these review processes dramatically curtailed PDT and other psychotherapeutic interventions.

These trends are grounded in a deep, long-standing societal stigma against patients with mental health conditions. The false perception that psychiatric patients are dangerous, murderous, gun-wielders remains a pervasive one in American society. At the same time, many Americans paradoxically minimize genuine complaints of feeling sadness or anxiety with careless comments such as "Quit bellyaching." In some horrifying instances, suicidal individuals have been egged on via text and social media to kill themselves.[23]

These negative images contribute to the collective societal perspective that, at worst, PDT is ineffective, nonempirical, out-of-date, and wasteful of time and money. Even at its best, the view of what PDT is; that is, its indications and its efficacy, is confused and uncertain. Insurance and pharmaceutical industries frequently perpetuate these negative stereotypes and confused preconceptions by defining psychiatrists as dispensers of medications, which best fits those institutions' models of care. Big Pharma can sell more medications if psychiatrists only prescribe and do not practice PDT; managed care organizations can cut costs if psychiatrists see patients only monthly for 15-minute medication checks.

Psychiatrists need to reclaim their identity as clinicians who treat the whole person. They need to resist definition by those corporate entities whose main incentive is financial gain for their shareholders, ahead of the provision of optimal health care to their patients.

PSYCHIATRISTS OFTEN DISCOUNT PUBLIC PERCEPTION

Despite the pervasive negativity and distorted public perception of psychiatrists and PDT, psychiatrists rarely defend themselves or their work.[24] However, public perception matters. Just consider how the recently minted concept of fake news affects political discourse today. Reasons for psychiatrists' passivity might include the following:

- Most psychiatrists seek the truth, and may tend to ignore or discount false perceptions, believing a response is not worth the effort.
- Research shows that some psychiatrists worry that focusing on their optics might be construed as attention-seeking and self-promotion.[25]
- In psychiatry, often, the learned, or normative, response to an attack is to contain the bad, rather than defend against it. Psychodynamic psychiatrists typically create a safe, holding environment in their therapeutic alliance with patients, and may be more comfortable with accepting and metabolizing false projections about themselves and their work than with defending themselves and proving the projection is wrong.

- Psychiatrists are also members of American society and have been exposed to societal stigma and influences; they may have unconsciously internalized and accepted these negative societal stereotypes and misperceptions.

WHY PSYCHIATRISTS SHOULD CARE ABOUT THE OPTICS OF PSYCHODYNAMIC THERAPY

PDT takes place within a complex web of multiple systems of care. Today, most of these systems are fraught with barriers that prevent patients from receiving the level or quality of care they need. Many of these systems are financially incentivized to limit access, which contains costs.[26] Most are intended to serve short-term goals, rather than make a long-term investment in patient mental health. It is important for psychiatrists to recognize that these systems interact and overlap to affect the quality and type of mental health care that patients receive. These systems include:

- The policies and procedures of psychiatric service systems, including hospitals, community mental health centers, outpatient clinics, and private practice offices
- Insurance and managed care organizations' guidelines
- Local, state, and federal laws and regulations
- Social determinants of health, such as socioeconomic status, gender, race, ethnicity, and age

Psychiatrists need to work to bring structural change to the current financial and regulatory framework of care in order to remove barriers to quality psychiatric care. They need to try to change public attitudes, which affect these systems. Psychiatrists also need to advocate to reclaim their dual identity as psychotherapists and medical providers, rather than allow health care industries to truncate their professional roles into mere diagnosticians and prescription dispensers. If psychiatrists do not act, these systems are unlikely to change.

ADVOCACY AND THE MEDICAL PROFESSION

Merriam-Webster defines an advocate as one who "pleads the cause of another" and "supports or promotes the interests of a cause or group." Advocates work to communicate information about an issue such that they educate and increase awareness in target audiences to effect change, including stakeholders, decision-makers, the media, and social media influencers.[27] Advocacy can focus on changing political, legal, social, and/or economic systems, and can be accomplished by individuals, groups, or coalitions of groups. Advocacy today is a highly sophisticated and complex social science that involves aspects of communication, semiotics, psychology, education, and sociology.

Advocacy can be motivated by values based in moral, ethical, or religious beliefs, or it can be driven by science and research.[28] Whatever the goal, advocates need to use specialized skills to be effective.

Key Advocacy Skills

Advocacy skills are not intuitive; they require training and practice. The verb skill originally meant "to make a difference," and an advocate's goal is to make a difference in how his or her issue is understood and perceived. In the medical profession, the advocacy skill set should include:

- The ability to conceptualize and frame issues to create a message
- The ability to translate research into clear concepts

- The ability to translate research and policy into action
- The ability to anticipate rebuttal arguments and have prepared responses on hand.

Effective advocacy also depends on excellent oral and written communication skills. Tools advocates use include:

- Speeches and interviews
- Letters, articles, and opinion pieces
- Policy briefs.

Advocates need effective teaching skills and the ability to target different audiences and tailor their messages to each specific audience, including:

- Legislators
- Regulators
- Media and social media influencers
- Medical professionals in different fields
- Nonmedical health care providers
- Patient advocacy groups
- The general public.

The job of the advocate is to:

- Identify key decision-makers and build relationships
- Promote public discourse
- Develop grassroots organizations
- Engage organizations to build coalitions.

The Physician's Duty to Advocate

The American Medical Association (AMA) asserts in its "Declaration of Professional Responsibility" that "physicians commit themselves to…advocate for social, economic, educational, and political changes that ameliorate suffering and contribute to well-being." The Board of Trustees for the American Psychiatric Association (APA) also ratified this professional obligation for psychiatrists to advocate for issues that help patients.

Physicians have successful track records as advocates. For example, pediatricians spearheaded a children's safety-seat campaign; today, all 50 states require children to travel in cars with approved safety restraints. Dr Luther Terry, US Surgeon General, chose to broadly publicize the link between cigarettes and lung cancer; this effort led to dramatically lower smoking rates within a generation and averted nearly 800,000 deaths from lung cancer.[29]

In general, physicians are especially well-equipped to advocate for their patients. As noted in the Gallup Poll, physicians are viewed positively by society and are seen as:

- Highly educated, able to understand complexity
- Rooted in an evidence-based orientation
- Objective, unbiased, and trustworthy
- Authoritative and deserving of respect
- Speaking from first-hand experience, with patient stories to offer
- Able to translate research data into policy and messaging.

These favorable perceptions have enabled physician advocacy and led to important social, legal, and attitudinal changes within American society. Physicians can advocate independently, or through their affiliations with professional organizations, such as the AMA and APA, or through an issues-oriented campaign.

A Campaign Model

A campaign is an organized effort that includes clearly defined goals, a candidate, a consistent message, a target group or groups, and a strategic plan for grassroots engagement and coalition-building. Every campaign is unique and must constantly evolve to respond to external challenges and demands.[30]

A campaign must thoughtfully and carefully design an effective message that will be repeated over and over again. This message must be clear and powerful, and it must not reinforce or incite resistance and opposition. Repetition cannot be overemphasized. Advertising research suggests that multiple touches from a variety of sources will eventually lead to an incorporation of the message by the target audience.[31,32]

The purpose of any campaign is to emotionally motivate the target audience to choose the campaign's candidate over others. Although other candidates may be superficially more gratifying (smoking), or require less effort (not bothering with child safety restraints), an effective campaign will find a way to promote its candidate regardless of intrinsic impediments. Today, most Americans choose not to smoke and most parents choose to use child safety restraints.

A CAMPAIGN FOR PSYCHODYNAMIC THERAPY

Imagine how psychiatrist-advocates might design the first steps of a campaign for PDT. The candidate would be PDT, and the initial steps toward a successful campaign would include identifying the strengths and weaknesses of the candidate, identifying the opposition and its weaknesses, crafting an effective message, identifying the target audiences, and building a grassroots coalition. All of these steps would have the purpose of implementing the list of designated campaign goals and corresponding action plans, as shown in **Table 1**.

The Candidate's Strengths and Weaknesses

Every campaign needs to take stock of the strengths and weaknesses of the candidate. This should be done from an objective perspective, ideally through the lens of the opposition. Advocates in a campaign for PDT might list the following strengths:

- Effective
- Cost-effective
- Safe; no medication side effects.

Weaknesses for PDT might include that it is:

- Perceived as noneffective and lacking empirical data to support its efficacy
- Considered too costly; more expensive than medication
- Wasteful, empty talk
- Out-of-date, not modern
- Difficult to explain; filled with vague concepts and jargon
- Without a concrete, positive, visual representation
- Already viewed negatively; it is difficult to overcome intrinsic bias and change opinions once formed.

Subsequent steps would be to reframe these weaknesses as strengths, and convey these to advocates to help them anticipate and rebut attacks and criticisms.

Identify and Reframe the Weaknesses of the Opponents

Advocates for PDT need to pinpoint forces in the healthcare delivery system that undermine PDT and conceptualize these forces as "opponents." Then, advocates

Table 1
Campaign goals and action plan

Goals	Action Plan
Change the general public's perception of PDT	Deploy opinion pieces in online and print news publications Get earned media to convey message Seed social media and pop culture with positive images and references about PDT Engage grassroots groups, especially social media influencers, to share message on social media Engage celebrities to broadcast testimonials about the power of PDT
Change general psychiatrists' perception of PDT	Change research funding metrics to continue to build an evidence base for psychotherapy Conduct workshops and educational seminars
Change nonpsychiatrists' perception of PDT	Build coalitions and gain support from a range of nonpsychiatric medical organizations, including APA and AMA Conduct workshops and educational seminars
Change insurance and reimbursement systems that constrain the practice of PDT	Respond vigorously to all denials of care Notify state insurance commissioner of inconsistencies If necessary, engage attorneys
Ensure that parity, as defined by the Mental Health Parity and Addiction Equity Act, is enforced	Monitor federal regulations and engage federal legislators to change, if necessary Monitor state regulations and engage state legislators to change, if necessary Work with APA
Ensure that psychiatry residency training programs are teaching PDT	Engage American Association of Directors of Psychiatric Residency Training to review programs

should do opposition research on these opponents in order to determine strengths and potential vulnerabilities. Identified strengths should be reframed in ways that weaken the opponent and/or benefit PDT.This reframing should feel authentic and relatable to the target audiences. Advocates should not dredge up (or worse, manufacture) scandals because the purpose is not to discredit or devalue the opponent per se. Rather, advocates need to underscore the differences between their candidate and the opponents.

Craft an Effective Message

A campaign message should have the goal of promoting, educating, and inspiring its target audience. In the case of PDT, crafting an effective message is a challenge. PDT is inherently conceptual, difficult to explain, and confusing; and it lacks concrete physical characteristics. The message should not incite backlash and further criticism; advocates should not launch attacks on the pharmaceutical ("Stop excessive psychopharmacology") or insurance industries ("Insurance companies are greedy").

PDT has already been widely defined negatively and its image requires reframing, which requires careful thought.[33] Messaging for PDT should aim to dispel inaccurate perceptions through evidence-based messaging[34] that targets efficacy, cost-effectiveness, and safety. Messaging should be built on a foundation of scientific studies and evidence-based research. The message should:

- Be clear and concise
- Present scientific evidence but not use scientific jargon
- Be geared to the target audience.

Identify the Target Audiences

Advocates will need to identify their target audiences so that they can tailor their advocacy activities to that audience, taking into account the specific target audience's intrinsic biases, education, culture, motivations, and concerns. In advocacy for PDT, target audiences might include:

- Medical students; psychiatry residents and fellows
- Non-PDT psychiatrists; nonpsychiatrist physicians
- Nonmedical health care providers
- Health care administrators
- Health care investors
- Federal and private organizations that fund research
- Professional societies and organizations
- Community organizations with a mental health focus
- Patient advocacy organizations
- Traditional media outlets, including print, radio, television, and film
- Social media influencers
- State and federal legislators, administrators, and regulators
- The general public.

Organize Grassroots Groups and Build Coalitions

Advocates can start at the local and community levels, educating fellow physicians and nonphysicians about the efficacy of PDT. They can also work within their professional organizations, such as state medical and psychiatric societies, to change perceptions about PDT. Advocates may consider reaching out to local chapters of patient organizations, such as the National Alliance on Mental Illness.

Advocates need to work toward more accurate representations of PDT in the media, including print, radio, television, and film. Advocates will need to find creative ways to promote PDT to the general public, based on the characteristics of the target audience. In today's world, most people would not be inspired or moved by an advertisement of a tearful patient sitting in an oversized armchair next to a concerned therapist.

Advocates should consider novel promotional methods to reach new target audiences to build grassroots organizations.[35] Advocates could focus on identifying and engaging potential social media influencers whose social media presence is substantial; for example, one who has more than 100,000 Twitter followers. Is there the equivalent of a Taylor Swift or LeBron James for the promotion of PDT?

Building grassroots organizations and coalitions at any level requires advocates to tailor their message to the target audience. Including the following elements can enhance any presentation focused on grassroots engagement:

- Present compelling vignettes
- Be credible; do not make inauthentic statements
- Identify the results of inaction

- Suggest specific action by the target audience to ensure engagement; that is, sign a petition, join an email listserve, or follow on social media
- Anticipate criticism and be prepared with nondefensive responses.

Define the Timeline

Whereas political campaigns have defined endings (Election Day) a multisystem campaign for PDT has an open-ended timeline with a far-off horizon.

PSYCHIATRIST ADVOCACY FOR PSYCHODYNAMIC THERAPY

Regardless of whether a campaign is organized, advocacy for PDT can take many forms. Legislative advocacy focuses on changing laws and regulations at the local, state, and federal level that may impede access to PDT. Legal advocacy focuses on helping patients obtain legal remedies to overly restrictive insurance carriers' guidelines that disregard parity and deny PDT. Research advocacy focuses on reversing the negative bias against the funding of PDT research. Attitudinal advocacy focuses on changing attitudes and perceptions in various populations, including the general public, psychiatric patients, general psychiatrists, and nonpsychiatric physicians. Advocacy for PDT should not be construed as political speech and should aim for a nonpartisan approach.

Psychiatrists can be the strongest advocates for PDT, despite being hampered by negative stereotypes and false perceptions about PDT by the public at large. Psychiatrists are the professionals who can best present empirical data about the benefits of PDT, and have the relationship skills to connect with their target audiences. Psychiatrists can advocate in a variety of ways. They can:

- Work within their institutions to change how clinical services are organized and remunerated
- Lobby within a professional organization to promote an accurate understanding of PDT
- Lobby on behalf of a professional organization
- Lead or develop a grassroots organization
- Educate patients, other professionals, and/or the general public about the benefits of PDT
- Monitor managed care companies for inadequate provider networks, improper treatment denials, and parity violations; and facilitate legal action if necessary
- Advocate to improve state and federal laws around insurance regulations and reimbursement policies
- Advocate for funding to support PDT research.

Specific actions psychiatrists can take to advocate for PDT:

- If a patient's treatment preauthorization is denied, respond, be persistent, and bring legal action if necessary, and, for future reference, maintain a record of the denial
- Educate medical colleagues, both psychiatric and nonpsychiatric, either in formal presentations or informal curbside chats, about the safety, efficacy, and cost-effectiveness of PDT
- If inadequate insurance provider networks are identified, bring the issue to the attention of state insurance regulators
- Monitor for parity violations of state and federal regulations; if indicated, bring violations to the attention of regulators and lawmakers
- Understand current state and federal insurance legislation; if inadequate, bring the problem to the attention of lawmakers

- Volunteer for a local, state, or federal campaign for a legislator who favors PDT; a psychiatrist's role can range from knocking on doors to providing research for policy position statements
- Develop relationships with state legislators and brief them about the benefits of PDT
- Educate the general public via op-eds and letters to the editor of local and national media
- Identify media and social media influencers and engage them to spread positive messages and images about the benefits of PDT
- Educate supervisees and students about the benefits of PDT
- Make sure the area psychiatry residency training program has a robust curriculum for training residents in PDT skills
- If a member of the APA, join the Psychotherapy Caucus by emailing ssugarman@psych.org
- If a member of the APA, consider joining the Congressional Advocacy Network and supporting the APA Political Action Committee; although neither directly advocates for PDT, both provide support and advocacy for issues of importance to PDT, such as parity, network adequacy, and research.

WHAT ARE THE CHALLENGES TO EFFECTIVE ADVOCACY?

Advocacy work is challenging, regardless of the issue. It is hard work, it takes time, and it exacts costs on advocates. Any advocate might face 1 or all of the following challenges.

General Challenges to Effective Advocacy

- Lack of time: No matter how large or small the issue, advocacy efforts demand time, a scarce commodity for most people, whether campaigning to stop global warming or to install a stoplight on a dangerous corner.
- Logistical issues: The logistics of advocacy efforts, including the scheduling for both planned activities and unexpected demands, may not fit easily into advocates' routines, especially if their schedules lack flexibility. For example, an all-day public hearing might be publicized with only 72 hours' notice; canceling work-related appointments at such short notice may be difficult.
- Lack of training in advocacy skills: Many advocates may feel uncomfortable with advocacy tasks, such as public speaking, social media communications, and written communications such as opinion pieces and petitions. To execute these advocacy tasks effectively, advocates need training and mentoring.
- Isolation: Many advocates can feel alone, as if in a solitary fight for their cause. Advocacy thrives when there is a supportive community; this may explain why advocates favor marches and rallies: besides raising public awareness, these communal activities create a sense of solidarity and support.
- Hopelessness and burnout: Advocacy efforts can be frustrating, with unforeseen barriers, unexpected harsh criticism, and even vicious attacks. When advocacy timelines are long-term, with distant goals requiring years, and even decades to achieve, some advocates may develop feelings of hopelessness, find themselves unable to persevere, and experience burnout.

Psychiatrists who advocate for PDT face these challenges, as well as additional personal and professional challenges.

Challenges to Effective Advocacy by Psychiatrists Advocating for Psychodynamic Therapy

- Professional identity does not include advocacy: Despite AMA expectations that physicians act as advocates, few psychiatrists receive advocacy training during their residencies. They may experience difficulty integrating the advocacy role into their professional identity.
- Few psychiatrist role models: There are few seasoned psychiatrist-advocates with the experience to serve as role models, mentors, and teachers for new psychiatrist-advocates.
- Stigma: The negative attitudes toward psychiatrists among the general public and other groups are likely to create obstacles. For example, a psychiatrist may not be taken as seriously as a nonpsychiatric physician.
- Work–life balance and self-care: Psychiatrists' limited time resources are already allocated to tasks such as clinical care, professional development, administrative demands, supervision, teaching, and research. The time needed to develop advocacy skills may take away from time needed for wellness and self-care.
- Self-motivations for advocacy: Psychiatrists should question the reasons underlying their interest in advocacy. Does the interest stem from personal needs; that is, to fill empty time after a divorce or loss? Or from professional needs to advance one's career, enhance one's reputation, or gain publicity?
- Risk of malignant altruism or well-intended advocacy: Do advocacy efforts perform defensive functions; that is, does the psychiatrist enter into advocacy as a way of displacing other conflicts, either professional or personal?
- Discomfort with larger, more public media presence: Some psychiatrists may be uncomfortable with establishing a higher media profile and/or social media presence.
- Distaste for social media: Some psychiatrists may have a distaste for social media, and they may find including social media in their advocacy efforts especially onerous.
- Lack of systems training: Psychiatrists who were not trained with a systems model perspective may find it hard to conceptualize how to advocate to change systems of care.
- Difficulty balancing reflective and action-oriented work: Psychiatrists may find it hard to switch back and forth between the reflective and introspective work of psychotherapy and the action-oriented salesman type approach of advocacy.
- Tension between neutrality and expressing opinions: Psychiatrists may find it difficult to balance neutrality as a psychotherapist with the requirement to express opinions publicly as an advocate.

Potential Impacts of Advocacy to Clinical Work

In addition to the challenges, psychiatrists should evaluate whether advocacy might affect their clinical work. Psychiatrists should consider the potential of opportunity costs: the risk that passion for a cause detracts from clinical encounters. Psychiatrists might find that there are instances when the work of advocacy diminishes their capacity for self-reflection or affective engagement with patients. For example, the urgency of an advocacy demand may interfere with a psychiatrist's ability to be fully present during a therapeutic encounter.

Psychiatrists should consider their advocacy work when they reflect on the complex dynamics of their relationships with patients. Patients may be aware of their psychiatrist's advocacy efforts and may respond, either consciously or unconsciously, with signs of ambivalence, conflict, or resistance. Psychiatrists should be on the lookout for increased symptoms, a change in affect and/or the quality of material presented during a session, and avoidant or passive-aggressive behaviors, such as missed or canceled meetings, lateness attending appointments, and changes in the established payment protocol. Patients may also respond with unusual requests, gifts, or other acting-out or boundary-crossing behaviors. Psychiatrists need to monitor the treatment to determine whether outside advocacy efforts are affecting the therapy in a way that impedes progress or fosters resistance. If so, psychiatrists should address these behaviors therapeutically.

For psychiatrists engaged in advocacy, tolerating negative transferences may be challenging. Fighting on the advocacy front may take away from the energy required to hold and manage a negative transference, and the psychiatrist-advocate may feel increasingly beleaguered. Managing primitively organized patients' attacks may become harder. Psychiatrists should be alert to their own newly developed blind spots and countertransference responses.

Psychiatrists should also be aware of overly positive, idealizing transferences. Some patients may overvalue the psychiatrist's advocacy work, and withhold criticism or shield the therapist from their negative effects. Other patients may imagine the psychiatrist as a savior or powerful crusader who will also fight for them.

Psychiatrists need to consider their motivations when disclosing or discussing their advocacy efforts to patients, especially those who are themselves health care professionals or advocates. What is the underlying purpose of involving the patient in one's advocacy efforts? At the same time, psychiatrists should be careful not to collude with patients and avoid talking about advocacy. In general, the psychiatrist should explore requests and their meaning.

Finally, as in all work with patients, psychiatrists need to give careful attention to guidelines in the Health Insurance Portability and Accountability Act (HIPAA). Regard for confidentiality and potential ethical issues should underlie all therapeutic and advocacy work. In general, in clinical work, psychiatrist-advocates will need to:

- Integrate advocacy efforts into personal identity and work as a psychiatrist
- Be alert to potential transference or countertransference issues
- Explore fantasies and defenses that might arise in patients by the advocacy role
- Look for and monitor resistance
- Be constantly mindful of HIPAA guidelines and potential ethical conflicts.

SUMMARY

Advocating for PDT presents challenges for psychodynamic psychiatrists and (perhaps) some unanticipated rewards, such as new skills, new colleagues, and (possibly) success. Psychiatrists need to advocate for attitudinal shifts and financial and regulatory system change for PDT, so that patients can better access this safe, effective, and cost-effective mental health treatment. To ensure that PDT exists in the future American health care system, psychiatrists should start to advocate today.

REFERENCES

1. Bendat M. In name only? Mental health parity or illusory reform. Psychodyn Psychiatry 2014;42:353–75.
2. Abbass A, Luyten P, Steinert C, et al. Bias toward psychodynamic therapy: framing the problem and working toward a solution. J Psychiatr Pract 2017;23:363–5.

3. Stuart H, Sartorius N, Liinamaa T, the Images Study Group. Images of psychiatry and psychiatrists. Acta Psychiatr Scand 2015;131:21–8.
4. Clemens N, Plakun E, Lazar S, et al. Obstacles to early career psychiatrists practicing psychotherapy. Psychodyn Psychiatry 2014;42:479–96.
5. Levy K, Ehrenthal JC, Yeomans FE, et al. The efficacy of psychotherapy: focus on psychodynamic psychotherapy as an example. Psychodyn Psychiatry 2014;42: 377–421.
6. Leichsenring F, Rabung S, Leibing E. The efficacy of short-term psychodynamic psychotherapy in specific psychiatric disorders: a meta-analysis. Arch Gen Psychiatry 2004;61:1208–16.
7. Shedler J. The efficacy of psychodynamic psychotherapy. Am Psychol 2010;65: 98–109.
8. Steinert C, Munder T, Rabung S, et al. Psychodynamic therapy: as efficacious as other empirically supported treatments? A meta-analysis testing equivalence of outcomes. Am J Psychiatry 2017;174:943–53.
9. Huhn M, Tardy M, Spineli LM, et al. Efficacy of pharmacotherapy and psychotherapy for adult psychiatric disorders: a systematic overview of meta-analysis. JAMA Psychiatry 2014;71:706–15.
10. Cuijpers P, Sijbrandij M, Koole SL, et al. Adding psychotherapy to antidepressant medication in depression and anxiety disorders: a meta-analysis. World Psychiatry 2014;13:56–67.
11. Tasman A, Riba MB. Psychological management in psychopharmacologic treatment, and combination pharmacologic and psychotherapeutic treatment. In: Lieberman JA, Tasman A, editors. Psychiatric drugs. Philadelphia: WB Saunders Company; 2000. p. 242–9.
12. Miklowitz D. Adjunctive psychotherapy for bipolar disorder: State of the evidence. Am J Psychiatry 2008;165:1408–19.
13. Abbass A, Hancock JT, Henderson J, et al. Short-term psychodynamic psychotherapies for common mental disorders. Cochrane Database Syst Rev 2006;(4):CD004687.
14. Lazar S. Psychotherapy is worth it: a comprehensive review of its cost-effectiveness. Washington, DC: American Psychiatric Publishing, Inc; 2010.
15. Lazar S. The cost-effectiveness of psychotherapy for the major psychiatric diagnoses. Psychodyn Psychiatry 2014;42:423–58.
16. Linden M. How to define, find and classify side effects in psychotherapy: from unwanted events to adverse treatment reactions. Clin Psychol Psychother 2013; 20(4):286–96.
17. ACGME Program Requirements for Graduate Medical Education in Psychiatry. Available at: https://www.acgme.org/Portals/0/PFAssets/ProgramRequirements/400_psychiatry_2017-07-01.pdf. Accessed October 20, 2017.
18. Wipond R. Psychiatrists discuss psychiatry's poor public image and what to do about it. 2014. Available at: https://www.madinamerica.com/2014/12/psychiatrists-discuss-psychiatrys-poor-public-image/. Accessed October 17, 2017.
19. Gaebel W, Zielasek J. Overcoming stigmatizing attitudes towards psychiatrists and psychiatry. Acta Psychiatr Scand 2015;131:5–7.
20. Honesty/ethics in professions. Gallup News 2016. Available at: http://news.gallup.com/poll/1654/honesty-ethics-professions.aspx. Accessed November 2, 2017.
21. Psychiatrists and psychologists: understanding the differences. 2016. Available at: https://www.psychiatry.org/news-room/apa-blogs/apa-blog/2016/02/psychiatrists-and-psychologists-understanding-the-differences. Accessed November 7, 2017.

22. Claridge JA, Fabian TC. History and development of evidence-based medicine. World J Surg 2005;29(5):547–53.
23. Woman sentenced to 15 months in texting suicide case. 2017. Available at: http://www.cnn.com/2017/08/03/us/michelle-carter-texting-suicide-sentencing/index.html. Accessed November 5, 2017.
24. Lamontagne Y. The public image of psychiatrists. Can J Psychiatry 1990;35:693–5.
25. Shonkoff JP, Bales SN. Science does not speak for itself: translating child development research for the public and its policy makers. Child Dev 2011;82:17–32.
26. Plakun E. Psychotherapy, parity and ethical utilization management. J Psychiatr Pract 2017;23:49–52.
27. Division of Health Education. Advocacy strategies for health and development: development communication in action. Geneva (Switzerland): World Health Organization; 1992. Available at: http://apps.who.int/iris/bitstream/10665/70051/1/HED_92.4_eng.pdf. Accessed November 6, 2017.
28. Farrer L, Marinetti C, Kuipers Caraco Y, et al. Advocacy for health equity: a synthesis review. Milbank Q 2015;93:392–437.
29. Moolgavkar SH, Holford TR, Levy DT, et al. Impact of reduced tobacco smoking on lung cancer mortality in the United States during 1975-2000. J Natl Cancer Inst 2012;104(7):541–8.
30. Guzzetta SJ. The campaign manual: a definitive study of the modern political campaign process. Deer Park (NY): Linus Publications; 2006.
31. Lynn S. Political campaign planning manual for the National Democratic Institute for International Affairs. Available at: https://www.ndi.org/sites/default/files/Political_Campaign_Planning_Manual_Malaysia_0.pdf. Accessed October 29, 2017.
32. Martic GJ, Yurukoglu A. Bias in cable news: persuasion and polarization. 2017. Available at: https://web.stanford.edu/~ayurukog/cable_news.pdf. Accessed November 2, 2017.
33. Dorfman L, Wallack L, Woodruff K. More than a message: framing public health advocacy to change corporate practices. Health Educ Behav 2005;32:320–36.
34. Friedlaender E, Winston F. Evidence based advocacy. Inj Prev 2004;10:324–6.
35. Madia S. The social media survival guide for political campaigns. Voorhees (NJ): Full Court Press; 2011.

Innovative Educational Initiatives to Train Psychodynamic Psychiatrists in Underserved Areas of the World

César A. Alfonso, MD[a,b,*], Marco Christian Michael, MD, BMedSc[c], Sylvia Detri Elvira, MD[c], Hazli Zakaria, MBBS[b], Rasmon Kalayasiri, MD[d], Aida Syarinaz A. Adlan, MBBS, MPM[e], Mahdieh Moinalghorabaei, MD[f], Petrin Redayani Lukman, MD, MMedEd[g], Mohammad San'ati, MD[f], Katerina Duchonova, MD[h], Timothy B. Sullivan, MD[h,i]

KEYWORDS

• Psychodynamic psychiatry • Psychotherapy • Transcultural psychiatry
• Psychiatric education • Low-income and middle-income countries

KEY POINTS

- Psychotherapy training is insufficient despite available standardized psychiatric residency curricula.
- Cultural adaptations of psychotherapy remain crucial and relevant in psychiatric training.
- Pedagogical innovations with international collaborations bridge educational gaps of psychodynamic psychiatrists in underserved countries.

Disclosure Statement: The authors have disclosed that they have no financial conflict of interest with any manufacturer of commercial products or services.

[a] Department of Psychiatry, Columbia University Medical Center, 1051 Riverside Drive, New York, NY 10032, USA; [b] Department of Psychiatry, National University of Malaysia, Jalan Yacob Latiff, Cheras, Kuala Lumpur 56000, Malaysia; [c] Department of Psychiatry, Universitas Indonesia, Jl. Kimia II No 35, Jakarta Pusat, DKI Jakarta 10430, Indonesia; [d] Department of Psychiatry, Chulalongkorn University, 1873 Rama 4 Road, Pathumwan, Bangkok 10330, Thailand; [e] Department of Psychological Medicine, University of Malaya, Lembah Pantai, Kuala Lumpur 50603, Malaysia; [f] Department of Psychiatry, Tehran University of Medical Sciences, No. 606, South Kargar Street, District 11, Tehran, Iran; [g] Department of Psychiatry, Military University Hospital Prague, U Vojenske nemocnice 1200, Prague 169 02, Czech Republic; [h] Department of Psychiatry, Hofstra Northwell SOM, 376 Seguine Avenue, Staten Island, NY 10309, USA; [i] Department of Behavioral Sciences, Hofstra Northwell SOM, 376 Seguine Avenue, Staten Island, NY 10309, USA

* Corresponding author. 262 Central Park West, Suite #1B, New York, NY 10024.
E-mail address: caa2105@cumc.columbia.edu

Psychiatr Clin N Am 41 (2018) 305–318
https://doi.org/10.1016/j.psc.2018.01.010 psych.theclinics.com
0193-953X/18/

INTRODUCTION

Although psychoanalysis is not commonly practiced in many areas of the world, psychodynamic perspectives and constructs enhance the standard of care of the more widely used supportive and cognitive-behavioral (CBT) psychotherapies. The multimodal integrative approach of balancing cognitive restructuring and correcting cognitive distortions, along with uncovering, interpretative, and supportive interventions, helps patients understand behavior and gain higher levels of functioning.

This article describes educational initiatives of the World Psychiatric Association (WPA) in collaboration with psychiatrists in Thailand, Indonesia, and Malaysia; and a psychotherapy training fellowship in Iran that emphasizes psychodynamic theory. Educators who are officers and members of the WPA sections (committees) on Psychoanalysis in Psychiatry and Education in Psychiatry and Psychotherapy, from Columbia University, Chulalongkorn University, the Royal College of Psychiatrists in Thailand, the Universitas Indonesia, University of Malaya, and the National University of Malaysia, designed a teaching and mentoring program to improve competency in psychodynamic psychotherapy.[1] The WPA project included a series of live workshops, followed by a semester of advanced psychotherapy courses using video conferencing and email moderated discussions, with the objective to train psychiatrists to become expert psychotherapists. Additionally, faculty development seminars were designed to engage course graduates to develop pedagogical skills. Also, a mentoring system was created to ensure self-sufficiency and enduring results. The Tehran University of Medical Sciences (TUMS) Psychotherapy Fellowship Program is also presented as an alternative advanced psychotherapy educational model that could be replicated in other countries.

Challenges affecting the implementation of educational models include limited psychiatric staffing resources, fulfilling public health needs, and considering cultural adaptations in psychotherapy training.

PSYCHIATRIC STAFFING RESOURCES WORLDWIDE

Worldwide, psychiatric staffing resources are influenced by income disparities. Staffing is of essence to provide adequate clinical services, as well as allowing more flexibility for physicians to balance academia with clinical duties.[2] Currently, the psychiatry workforce rate in the world is 1.2 per 100,000 (psychiatrists per 100,000 population, with an SD of 6.07), although psychiatrists are vastly unequally distributed. Europe has 9.8 per 100,000 and the United States 15.2 per 100,000, whereas Africa has approximately 1800 psychiatrists to take care of a population of greater than 700 million (0.04/100,000). The 2 most populous countries in the world, China and India, have estimated rates of 1.53 per 100,000 and 0.3 per 100,000, respectively. The World Health Organization (WHO) Global Health Observatory (GHO) 2015 data[3] needs to be interpreted with caution because it tends to underreport.[4]

The World Bank classifies countries into 4 categories based on income. Using the gross national income (GNI) per capita as an economic indicator, low-income, lower middle-income, upper-middle-income, and high-income countries are defined as those with GNI per capita of $1005 or less, $1006 to $3955, $3956 to $12,235, and $12,236 or more, respectively. This article focuses on countries with low-income or lower-middle-income economies because 149 out of 195 countries in the world are in this category. In these countries, the workforce disparities are overwhelming because 10% of the global psychiatric labor force cares for two-thirds of the world population.[4]

It is customary for specific geographic subregions to be consolidated as cultural zones determined by economic or other sociocultural agreements or clusters, such as the Association of South East Asian Nations (ASEAN) or Latin America. Notably, the cultural diversity between the nations included in these zonal conglomerates and that clinical reality psychiatrists face in the subregions varies widely. **Table 1** examines the psychiatric workforce diversity in the ASEAN and Latin America regions.

Table 1
Psychiatrists in Association of South East Asian Nations and Latin American countries

	GNI per Capita	Psychiatrists per 100,000 Population
Brunei	High	6
Cambodia	Lower-middle	0.34[32]
Indonesia	Lower-middle	0.29
Laos	Lower-middle	0.03
Malaysia	Upper-middle	0.8
Myanmar	Lower-middle	0.29
Philippines	Lower-middle	0.46
Singapore	High	3.48
Thailand	Upper-middle	0.87
Vietnam	Lower-middle	0.91
	GNI per Capita	**Psychiatrists per 100,000 Population**
Argentina	High	11.5
Bolivia	Lower-middle	0.82[32]
Brazil	Upper-middle	3.49
Chile	High	4.66
Colombia	Upper-middle	2.53
Costa Rica	Upper-middle	0.98[32]
Cuba	Upper-middle	2.08[32]
Dominican Republic	Upper-middle	1.08
Ecuador	Upper-middle	1.09
El Salvador	Lower-middle	0.32[32]
Guatemala	Lower-middle	0.29
Haiti	Low-income	0.07
Honduras	Lower-middle	0.38
Mexico	Upper-middle	0.67
Nicaragua	Lower-middle	0.65[32]
Panama	Upper-middle	3.80
Paraguay	Upper-middle	2.00
Peru	Upper-middle	0.76
Puerto Rico	High	2.37[32]
Uruguay	High	11.35[32]
Venezuela	Upper-middle	0.7[32]

Data from World Health Organization (WHO), World Psychiatric Association (WPA). Atlas: psychiatric education and training across the world 2005. Geneva (Switzerland): World Health Organization; 2005.

Regardless of psychiatric workforce general statistics, the provision of intensive psychotherapies is limited in most countries and formal psychoanalytic and psychodynamic psychotherapy training is rarely available outside of countries with high-income economies. This article examines creative ways to fulfill psychodynamic psychiatry competencies and offer training in underserved areas of the world.

PSYCHOTHERAPY EDUCATION: COMPETENCY VERSUS PUBLIC HEALTH APPROACHES

Competency-Based Education

Competency-based learning has come to be seen as a preferred training model because of its emphasis on the acquisition of practical, clinical skills (as opposed to traditional, theory-based training), though it has largely been implemented only in countries with high-income economies. This model assumes that psychiatrists should have expertise in treating a range of mental disorders, as well as possessing specific fundamental clinical skills.[5] In the United States, the Milestones Project, a joint initiative of the Accreditation Council of Graduate Medical Education and the American Board of Psychiatry and Neurology, provides a framework for the progressive assessment of trainees focusing on competencies that include psychotherapy and, specifically, psychodynamic psychotherapy.[6]

The competency-based learning model in countries with low-income and middle-income economies is difficult to implement.[4] Psychiatry residents in underserved areas struggle to provide ethical care to a high volume of patients while simultaneously attending to educational needs. In these scenarios, faculty members in busy hospitals and clinics teach best through clinical demonstrations rather than in the classroom. The apprenticeship model of 1-to-1 faculty–trainee clinical supervision is highly useful with respect to some clinical learning but may not produce desired outcomes if staffing resources are inadequate and if pressing service needs preclude protected educational experiences.

Public Health Emphasis

In challenged geographic areas, psychiatrists engage in clinical management and consultation as active liaisons with primary care providers, and take on public health leadership responsibilities.[7] A public health emphasis may be more prudent in the clinical care of persons in countries with low-income and middle-income economies. An educational model that expands care from the individual to the community would be ethically appropriate to match resources with the high burden of disease.

Most public health–informed care delivery models, especially in low-income and middle-income countries, assume that psychiatrists have very limited time to provide direct clinical services and, instead, focus on oversight and administering resources. This is the model proposed by Patel[8,9] to best address the global burden of mental illness, based on successful public health initiatives around the world. Changing the historical role of the psychiatrist from that of direct caregiver to that of supervisor or consultant, while meeting some clinical needs, poses risks. Among those risks is the concern that a psychiatrist who practices very little, and who has had limited clinical experience, may be ill equipped to supervise, especially over time. The health teams in the public health model are to be composed of diverse workers who could deliver specific tasks under the guidance of or in collaboration with psychiatrists. Such interdisciplinary collaboration is certainly beneficial; however, when using this model in particular, most psychotherapeutic interventions are assigned to counselors with more limited training.[4]

A Combined Educational Approach

The authors take the position that the competency-based and public health-minded pedagogical approaches can be combined to inform curricular and training model design, and that both aims can accommodate psychotherapy training and supervision of psychiatric residents, including in countries with low-income and middle-income economies. In such a combined model, psychotherapy training and, specifically, psychodynamic psychotherapy training are seen as informing the psychiatrist's understanding of systems and group dynamics (useful in serving as a team leader), as well as providing the psychiatrist with a sound clinical base from which to provide meaningful and expert guidance to team members. Also, the psychiatrist would take on the responsibility for the most complex cases, often providing care to those individuals directly. Primary care providers and other mental health clinicians would still carry the larger burden of care in these health systems.[4]

Some of the most complex cases include patients with multiple comorbidities, including the concurrent presence of severe personality disorder, together with patterns of impulsivity, heightened risk of self-harm, and frequent decompensation. These patients have been shown to benefit from psychodynamic psychotherapy[10–12] and, because they tend to be high users of services,[11] appropriate expert treatment by a well-trained psychiatrist may over the longer term realize significant cost-savings, as well as relieving suffering and improving quality of life. The literature suggests that pharmacotherapy in these patients is of limited benefit unless integrated with psychotherapy.[10,11] Research demonstrating that a psychotherapy dose effect is relevant for complex conditions supports this assertion.[11,13]

Although there are a variety of models with which providers can work, psychodynamic psychotherapy training has been shown to provide the best structure for safe and ethical practice. The authors maintain, with confidence, that psychodynamic training is essential because it affords practitioners the requisite skills to creatively adapt methodologies to the patient's circumstances while grounding the clinician in a framework that demands self-reflective awareness; attention to nuances of meaning and communication; and a profound, unwavering patient-centered focus. Because not all providers can be trained in psychodynamics, it is appropriate that the psychiatrist or team leader possess these skills.

The following sections describe examples of successful ongoing educational initiatives in diverse areas of the world, applying culturally informed models of collaborative care and competency-based approaches.

CULTURAL ADAPTATION OF PSYCHOTHERAPY TRAINING

Cultural adaptation of psychotherapy training addresses change over time; or the dynamics of societal, political, and other environmental factors that may influence the values and belief systems of individuals intergenerationally.

Understanding the cultural factors of the generational gaps between students and supervisors enhances the teaching processes in psychiatry.[14] In underserved areas, the competency-based training approach, although cumbersome if the psychiatric workforce is inadequate, may be increasingly plausible because younger trainees are more comfortable multitasking and can focus attention better than their teachers; they are highly skilled with swiftly shifting mental sets and can incorporate technological advances in learning and clinical practice. Nevertheless, sharing the burden of patient care with other mental health professionals may be prudent in underserved areas to optimize the use of scarce resources.

Psychiatry educators need to pay close attention to cultural factors associated with disease onset, illness course, and psychotherapy treatment outcomes. The biopsychosocial model postulates that the biomedical paradigm constricts clinical care, and exploration of psychosocial aspects is essential to be fully therapeutic.[15] Psychosocial determinants affect the therapeutic alliance, treatment adherence, treatment response, and prognosis.[16,17] Important psychosocial determinants in psychodynamic psychotherapy treatments include

- Understanding of illness
- Willingness to seek and accept treatment (ambivalence, contemplation, precontemplation)
- Shared attributes
- Learned attitudes
- Belief systems
- Value systems.

Societal and family views and attitudes about illness influence the psychotherapy discourse through transferences, enactments, and parallel processes.

Cultural sensitivity needs to take place beyond identifying relatively rare and exotic culture-bound syndromes, or encouraging trainees to mechanically construct cultural formulations. Although language affinity between clinician and patient promotes attunement, other factors are equally important. Determinants of cultural attunement include identifying

- Nuanced symbolic meaning that may be alien to the clinicians' way of thinking
- Idiosyncratic ways of communicating distress
- Idioms of distress that are culturally sanctioned or encouraged, such as a propensity toward either somatization or psychologizing, without fluid expression of affect.

Although, in the authors' collective experience, cultural similarities tend to outweigh differences, trainees need to understand the cultural makeup of each individual patient. The psychodynamic techniques of detailed inquiry and neutral curiosity[18] are helpful in constructing a careful anamnesis; however, this needs to occur without excessive countertransferential enthusiasm that could derail the process.

Of importance in psychotherapy training is exploration of cultural aspects of religion and spirituality in clinical care. It is challenging to incorporate cultural heritage data and the associated symbolism when making psychotherapeutic interpretations. Some basic knowledge of social sciences, such as philosophy, theology, and anthropology, could inform medical education and postgraduate training. Rather than assuming that spiritual advisers or community elders will contaminate the treatment space, psychotherapists should encourage synchronized efforts toward a common therapeutic goal. Creating liaisons with clergy, religious leaders, and organizations should be encouraged rather than discouraged, in the same way that collaborative models of care are inclusive of other health professionals.[4] Similarly, learning to be sensitive and neutral to historical and political development of different nations and ethnic groups, and their taboo themes could facilitate the development of the therapeutic alliance in transcultural treatments.

To adequately promote mental health, one needs to attend to the multiple dimensions of stigma as it relates to mental disorders in diverse populations. Other relevant cultural issues that permeate psychodynamic treatments include

- Attention to migration
- Traumatic displacement because of political turmoil

- The pandemic of intimate partner violence
- Victimization of children.

Learning to adequately liaise and advocate with social and protective services contextualizes psychotherapy treatments while protecting basic human rights.

TECHNOLOGY IN THE SERVICE OF BRIDGING EDUCATIONAL GAPS

Because incorporating technological advances in everyday life has taken on a life of its own, using the Internet in the practice of intensive psychotherapies is now widely accepted, despite pitfalls and legitimate concerns about protecting confidentiality. Similarly, Internet-based videoconferencing has been effectively used to bridge educational gaps in geographically compromised and underserved areas.[19]

The most successful distance learning enterprise is the China America Psychoanalytic Alliance (CAPA) educational programs, offering advanced psychodynamic psychotherapy courses, supervision, and personal psychotherapy to clinicians in China, mostly through secure Internet-based video with episodic site visits. More than 200 students have graduated from CAPA courses since its inception in 2008, and more than 150 volunteer faculty members from the Americas and Europe actively serve as educators.[20]

Other successful educational programs that are, at least in part, Internet-based include international collaborations between the University of Colorado School of Medicine and the University of Health Sciences Cambodia,[21] the Hamad Medical City Program in Qatar and Cornell University,[22] and the University of Toronto and Addis Ababa University in Ethiopia.[23] The following section details an innovative WPA intersectional program implemented in 3 ASEAN countries.

WORLD PSYCHIATRIC ASSOCIATION PSYCHODYNAMIC PSYCHOTHERAPY TRAINING PILOT PROGRAMS IN THE ASSOCIATION OF SOUTH EAST ASIAN NATIONS COUNTRIES

The aforementioned WPA sections identified a need to provide mentorship and facilitate career development in addition to offering workshops and symposia at regional conferences and world congresses. Psychiatrists, particularly from underserved areas, have a strong interest in learning psychodynamic psychotherapy. In Southeast Asia, young psychiatrists approached WPA speakers at regional conferences and asked for curricular guidance collaborations while clearly stating that clinical workshops were their preferred educational method for improving competency. As a result of this feedback, full-day workshops illustrating the relevance of psychodynamic thinking in a variety of clinical settings were piloted in Bangkok, Jakarta, and Surabaya beginning in 2012. An identical workshop was replicated in Kuala Lumpur during their national psychiatric conference in 2013.[24]

After preliminary planning in Bangkok in 2012, a pilot follow-up course was codesigned by colleagues from the Royal College of Psychiatrists of Thailand jointly with WPA section members, with the goal to train a select group of academic early-career Thai psychiatrists to improve their psychodynamic psychotherapy knowledgebase and gain confidence as clinical supervisors. The success of this course led to replication of the initiative in neighboring Malaysia and Indonesia. Over a period of 5 years, the WPA and national organizations in 3 ASEAN countries agreed to collaborate on a more comprehensive educational project. **Fig. 1** summarizes the 5-tiered pedagogical intervention now near completion.[1,25]

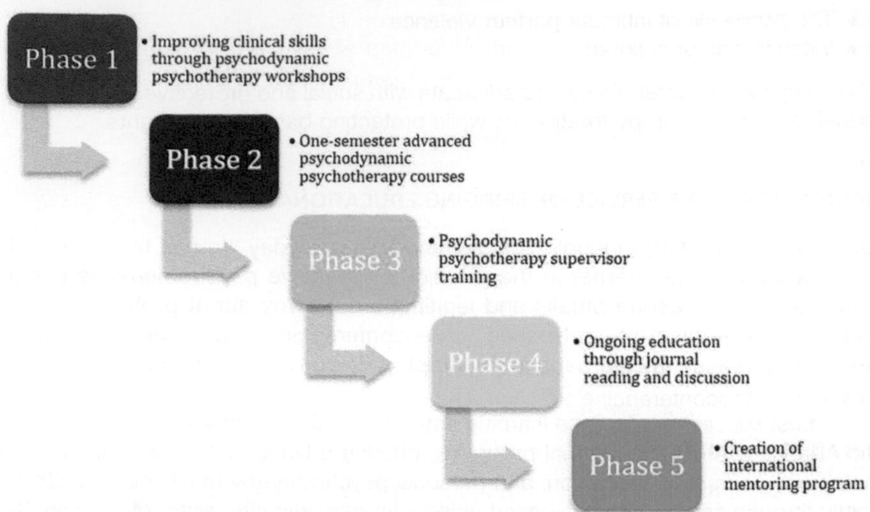

Fig. 1. Five-tiered pedagogical intervention.

Phase 1: Workshops to Improve Clinical Skills

Between 2012 and 2014, Alfonso, Zakaria, Aida Adlan, Kalayasiri, Elvira, and Lukman orchestrated multiple full-day advanced psychodynamic psychotherapy workshops in national meetings conducted by the Indonesian Psychiatric Association Psychotherapy Section in Jakarta and Surabaya, the Malaysian Psychiatric Association in Kuala Lumpur, and the Royal College of Psychiatrists of Thailand in Bangkok. WPA section chairs Tasman, Nahum, Botbol, Bennani, and WPA committee members Ammon and Onofrio were supportive of these efforts, because Asian countries at the time were underrepresented in the respective WPA sections.

Each workshop attracted approximately 35 to 50 participants; 260 participants attended the workshop in Kuala Lumpur. Local psychiatrists selected by host psychiatric societies ran these workshops and the modules were chosen according to the experts' areas of interest, with emphasis on application of psychodynamic thinking and clinical correlations in a variety of clinical settings. The local psychiatrists were invited to become active members of WPA sections or study groups on completion of the activities.[1]

Phase 2: 1-Semester Advanced Psychodynamic Psychotherapy Courses

Subsequently, for each of the 3 countries, a 1-semester follow-up advanced online psychodynamic psychotherapy course was designed and conducted sequentially over 2 years, in which 8 participants were chosen through a competitive application and selection process by the national societies. The course had a core curriculum of 40 selected articles and textbook chapters and was conducted mostly in a virtual classroom (90-minute class every other week through videoconference) in which peer and thematic supervision took place. A moderated email listserve discussion forum was established, as well as on-site learning at the end of the semester. The end of semester lesson was conducted in conjunction with the corresponding national psychiatric society meetings. The courses were held in 2014, 2015, and 2016, in Thailand, Malaysia, and Indonesia, respectively. Each course had 2 to 3 coteachers: César Alfonso (United States), Rasmon Kalayasiri (Thailand), Hazli Zakaria and Aida

Syarinaz Adlan (Malaysia), and Petrin Redayani Lukman and Sylvia Detri Elvira (Indonesia). In addition, the coteachers chose student-coordinators: Natchanan Charatcharungkiat (Thailand), Najwa Hanim Rosli (Malaysia), and Rizky Aniza Winanda (Indonesia).

The classes in this course were clinically focused in a case-conference style, in which each student was responsible for providing a written and oral presentation of a psychotherapy case, doing psychodynamic formulations, and preparing questions for discussion. Readings based on the core curriculum were matched based on the clinical relevance of individual cases, and students were required to critique theory and technique. To ensure engagement, classes were conducted bilingually in each respective country, while the student-coordinator served as the translator and maintained English as the common language. Patient confidentiality was protected by requesting informed consent, omitting identifying information, encrypting files, and using secure videoconferencing technologies.[1]

Phase 3: Training Psychodynamic Psychotherapy Supervisors

WPA intersectional leaders collaborated in designing full-day workshops aimed at improving supervision skills that took place in Indonesia and Malaysia. The first WPA intersectional workshop on psychodynamic psychotherapy supervision was in Malang, East Java, Indonesia, in March, 2017; the second was in Kuching, Sarawak, Malaysia, in July, 2017. These workshops were attended by a total of 75 participants, all psychiatrists engaged as intensive psychotherapy supervisors in academic medical centers. The workshops were also designed to further train the graduates of the phase 2 WPA psychodynamic psychotherapy programs to embrace their supervision responsibilities with mastery.

The supervision workshops combined small-group exercises and discussion, and brief lectures followed by interactive discussions. An interactive exercise examined the fine line between clinical supervision and psychotherapy of a supervisee, how to navigate between 1 dimension and the other, and under what circumstances one could integrate them in countries where residents have little or no access to their personal or training psychotherapy.

A workshop lecture module focused on describing psychodynamic psychotherapy competencies and ways to translate theory into technique through apprenticeship, including observation, collaboration, and assessment. Two videotapes were shown illustrating in vivo psychodynamic psychotherapy supervision, which highlighted how to teach theory and technique. Indonesian and Malaysian supervisors prepared these videos, which were conducted in Bahasa Indonesia with English subtitles and bilingually in Bahasa Melayu and English.

One workshop module focused in detail on the management of parallel processes in supervision, understanding enactments and projective counteridentification. Another module examined supervision as a process of progressive development, achieving mastery by moving along a continuum of milestones that progress from high motivation, inexperience, and high anxiety in beginners; fluctuating confidence and motivation with discouragement when facing impasses at midlevel; and security, consistency in attunement, serenity, and humility in advanced practice.[26]

A small-group exercise that followed focused on helping peers and trainees explore countertransferences in a systematic way, including erotic feelings and emotional states of boredom, rescue fantasies, rage, inadequacy, and sadness.

Finally, a workshop module traced the developmental progression of how supervisors help advance supervisees from inexperience to expertise, ego-supportively, by becoming self-objects and therapeutic role models. Workshop participants in this way learned how the transition from supervisors to mentors and peers brings about full circle the ultimate aim of clinical supervision.[1,27,28]

Phase 4: On-Going Education Through Review of Journal Readings

In the fall of 2017, graduates from the advanced course took charge of coordinating continuing education. Warut Aunjitsakul and Kanthee Anantapong, psychiatrists from Prince of Songkla University Thailand, coorganized of a 1-year psychotherapy journal club list serve for all 30 graduates and coteachers from the online courses. Activities of this phase include in-depth review of 12 recent articles published in the scientific journal *Psychodynamic Psychiatry*, in which an article is discussed every month over email list serve; journal article authors and editors are invited to mentor and participate in the discussions.[1]

Phase 5: Creating an International Mentoring Program

Course graduates and coteachers are also organizing an International Mentoring Association of Psychodynamic Psychiatrists, with the aim of advancing intensive psychotherapy practice through regional scientific meetings led by course graduates, and encouraging publications through collaborative efforts with WPA intersectional members serving as mentors and senior authors. This core group of mentors, teachers, and graduates is becoming a network of psychodynamic psychotherapy expert practitioners and supervisors.[1]

Although the long-term impact of this initiative is yet to be measured, since the inception of the pilot program, 15 graduates and all coteachers have actively participated in WPA-sponsored intersectional workshops and symposia in Hong Kong, China; Taipei, Taiwan; Berlin, Germany; and Florence, Italy, over the last triennium. They have published 3 articles in peer-reviewed journals, including *Psychodynamic Psychiatry*, the *ASEAN Journal of Psychiatry*, the *British Journal of Psychiatry International*, and contributed in 2 chapters to the upcoming edition of the book *Advances in Psychiatry*.[1,4,17,29,30]

In terms of overall program feedback, students appreciate the innovative educational approach that emphasizes group cohesion, as well as incorporating theory into practice. Difficulties such as complexity of the core curriculum and short deadline periods can be overcome by extending the course duration to allow additional time to discuss readings and increased coteacher presence during individual learning, while also providing sample video clips of experts conducting psychodynamic psychotherapy sessions.

Despite the perceived difficulty in providing psychodynamic training in countries with scarce resources, academics can make the most of current innovations in pedagogical methods by engaging in international collaborations with emphasis on mentorship and sensible cultural adaptations. With a directive of empowering and inspiring local talent, this educational model can perhaps be replicated in other underserved regions where psychotherapy training is suboptimal.

PSYCHODYNAMIC PSYCHOTHERAPY FELLOWSHIPS: THE TEHRAN UNIVERSITY OF MEDICAL SCIENCES MODEL

The Islamic Republic of Iran is located in Western Asia with an estimated population of 80 million as of 2017. Persia (Iran) has a rich medical history dating back millennia, as well as a strong psychiatric community with a psychotherapy tradition. Avicenna and Zakaraiyya al-Razi promoted the role of speech medicine and soul treatment as adjunctive to somatic treatments. The psychiatric workforce in Iran is mostly limited to the larger cities of Tehran, Isfahan, Mashhad, and Shiraz, where most of the 1700 Iranian psychiatrists practice in combined inpatient and outpatient settings. One of Iran's 14 university-based psychiatry residency training programs is the TUMS program, with 65 residents and 6 psychotherapy fellows. Political and economic sanctions imposed against Iran dating from 1979 resulted in marginalization and international seclusion from the academic community. Recently, some of the sanctions have eased and international participation in conferences, as well as videoconferencing, is beginning to reestablish Iranian psychiatry into the mainstream. The authors would like to highlight the psychotherapy fellowship program in TUMS for its comprehensiveness, attention to erudition, and clinical relevance.[4,31]

The TUMS psychotherapy fellowship is competitive and uncompromising. The fellowship emphasizes accepting trainees from diverse parts of Iran to equip them with the skills of becoming psychotherapy residency training supervisors. Through the 18-month program, early career psychiatrists or psychiatry residency graduates are allowed to learn through observation, assistance with and independent practice of psychodynamic psychotherapy, CBT, group psychotherapy, family therapy, spiritual psychotherapy, and supportive psychotherapy. In addition, enrollees work in treatment settings such as inpatient and outpatient psychiatric services (for 17 months), in conjunction with the psychosomatic medicine service (100 hours), child and adolescent psychiatry clinic (200 hours), addiction study center (100 hours), and a 1-month elective setting. San'ati developed a single-gender group therapy model that suits the Iranian socio-cultural context and is included in this fellowship program.[4,31]

At the end of the fellowship, trainees complete a total of

- 400 individual psychodynamic sessions
- 220 CBT sessions
- 70 schema therapy sessions
- 70 psychodynamic group psychotherapy sessions
- 42 CBT group psychotherapy sessions
- 60 family therapy sessions
- 1-month equivalency of spiritual therapies or 12 step-groups
- 24 sex therapy sessions
- 30 psychoeducation sessions.

The TUMS model uses didactic sources through 12 books (10 in English and 2 in Farsi) and 3 core journals: *International Journal of Psychoanalysis*, *American Journal of Psychotherapy*, and *International Journal of Psychotherapy*. The curriculum is flexible and individual teachers assign supplemental readings, with a high volume of reading materials covered in the span of the 18-month period. Trainees rely on primary sources with less dependence on textbooks, such as studying works by Freud, Klein, Fairbairn, Winnicott, Balint, Hartmann, Mahler, Jacobson, Spitz, Kernberg, Sandler, Mitchell, Lacan, Bowlby, and Adler, when they are studying psychodynamic psychiatry and learning the historical context of the development of other psychotherapies. The psychotherapy fellows also have responsibilities to teach medical and psychology students, as well as residents. In vivo observation and supervision are performed through 1-way mirror rooms or video camera recordings. Assessment of the program includes measurements of trainee satisfaction and feedback, level of satisfaction from faculty at universities that employ the graduates, and standardized faculty evaluations.[4,31]

Overall, The TUMS psychotherapy fellowship can be portrayed as an international model for rigorous training of advanced level psychiatry residents who are expected to take on teaching and supervisory responsibilities. San'ati and Moinalghorabaei, both UK-trained physicians, are teaching and training younger psychiatrists to become psychotherapy supervisors with emphasis on a high standard of care through combined and integrative psychotherapy methods. San'ati and Moinalghorabaei are psychoanalytically trained and place emphasis in teaching psychodynamic theories. As psychodynamic psychiatrists and educators, they encourage transtheoretical thinking and integrative practices, and help their trainees navigate with comfort as they become proficient with different psychotherapy modalities.[4,31]

SUMMARY

Although it may seem paradoxic that psychiatrists in underserved areas in low-income and middle-income countries are enthusiastic about learning psychodynamic theory and pursue training to advance intensive psychotherapy skills, on further reflection one realizes that the depth and breadth of psychodynamic training can serve organizing purposes by increasing the clinician's ego strength. A psychodynamic perspective also helps psychiatrists navigate through the complexity of imperfect systems with challenging public health needs. International collaborations that capitalize on principles of mentoring by providing self-object experiences are welcome and effective, especially under the umbrella of reputable organizations such as the WPA. Teachers, supervisors, and mentors are in a unique position to provide mirroring, idealizing, and twinship self-object experiences in an ego-supportive academic environment. The authors emphatically recommend maximizing the use of Internet technologies to bridge learning gaps. The authors favor condensed didactic interventions that highlight clinical relevance and correlation rather than the conventional, theory-heavy, lengthy postgraduate programs endorsed by psychoanalytic institutes in existence for more than a century in high-income countries. If the latter, conventional, Eurocentric model is preferred, the authors recommend shorter versions of integrated fellowship training templates such as the TUMS program. Finally, it is important to be mindful that all innovative didactic interventions should have as an aim to be self-sustaining, by training students to develop their own teaching and supervisory skills.

REFERENCES

1. Alfonso CAA, Sutanto L, Zakaria H, et al. Psychodynamic psychotherapy training in Southeast Asia—a distance learning pilot program. B J Psych Int 2018;15(1): 8–11.
2. Tasman A, Sartorius N, Saraceno B. Addressing mental health resource deficiencies in Pacific Rim countries. Asia Pac Psychiatr 2009;1:3–8.
3. WHO, WPA. Atlas: psychiatric education and training across the world. Geneva (Switzerland): World Health Organization; 2005.
4. Alfonso CA, Summers RF, Kronfol Z, et al. Psychiatry residency education in countries with low and middle-income economies. In: Fountolakis KN, Javed A, editors. Advances in psychiatry. Springer International Publishing, in press.
5. Casanova Dias M, Riese F, Tasman A. Curriculum development for psychiatric training. In: Fiorillo A, Volpe U, Bhugra D, editors. Psychiatry in practice: education, experience and expertise. Oxford (United Kingdom): Oxford University Press; 2016. p. 149–64.
6. Accreditation Council for Graduate Medical Education. The Psychiatry Milestone Project. 2015. Available at: https://www.acgme.org/Portals/0/PDFs/Milestones/PsychiatryMilestones.pdf. Accessed August 17, 2017.

7. Kigozi F, Ssebunnya J. The multiplier role of psychiatrists in low-income settings. Epidemiol Psychiatr Sci 2014;23:123–7.
8. Patel V. Mental health in low-and middle-income copuntries. Br Med Bull 2007;81: 81–96.
9. Patel V. The future of psychiatry in low-and middle-income countries. Psychol Med 2009;39:1759–62.
10. Levy KN, Ehrenthal JC, Yeomans FE, et al. The efficacy of psychotherapy: focus on psychodynamic psychotherapy as an example. Psychodyn Psychiatry 2014; 42(3):377–422.
11. Leichsenring F, Abbass A, Luyten P, et al. The emerging evidence for long-term psychodynamic therapy. Psychodyn Psychiatry 2013;41(3):361–84.
12. Fonagy P, Leigh SM, Steele H, et al. The relation of attachment status, psychiatric classification, and response to psychotherapy. J Consult Clin Psychol 1996;64: 22–31.
13. Howard KI, Kopta SM, Krause MS, et al. The dose–effect relationship in psychotherapy. Am Psychol 1986;41(2):159–64.
14. Beaglehole AL, Baig BJ, Stewart RC, et al. Training in transcultural psychiatry and delivery of education in a low-income country. Psychiatr Bull 2008;32:111–2.
15. Engel GL. The need for a new medical model: a challenge for biomedicine. Science 1977;196(4286):129–36.
16. Udomratn P. The assimilation of current Western psychotherapeutic practice in Thailand. IFP Newsletter 2008;6(1):13–15y.
17. Alfonso CA. Understanding the psychodynamics of non-adherence. Psychiatr Times 2011;28:22–3.
18. Sullivan HS. The psychiatric interview. New York: W.W. Norton & Co; 1958.
19. Hilty DM, Marks SL, Umess D. Clinical and educational telepsychiatry applications: a review. Can J Psychiatry 2004;11:35–8.
20. Fishkin R, Fishkin L, Leli U, et al. Psychodynamic treatment, training and supervision using internet-based technologies. J Am Acad Psychoanal Dyn Psychiatry 2011;39(1):155.
21. Savin DM, Kaur Legha R, Cordaro AR, et al. Spanning distance and culture in psychiatric education: a teleconferencing collaboration between Cambodia and the United States. Acad Psychiatry 2013;37(5):355–60.
22. Chouchane L, Mamtani R, Al-Thani MH, et al. Medical education and research environment in Qatar: a new epoch for translational research in the Middle East. J Transl Med 2011;9:16.
23. Alem A, Pain C, Araya M, et al. Co-creating a psychiatric resident program with Ethiopians, for Ethiopians, in Ethiopia: the Toronto Addis Ababa Psychiatry Project (TAAPP). Acad Psychiatry 2010;34:424–32.
24. Alfonso CA, Adlan ASA, Zakaria H, et al. Psychotherapy Training in Malaysia-Opportunities for improving competency through international collaboration. ASEAN J Psychiatry 2016;17(2):137–8.
25. Alfonso CA. Creating a psychodynamic psychotherapy-mentoring network and faculty development program in Southeast Asia—a 5-year pilot program, Proceedings of the 18th World Congress of the World Association of Dynamic Psychiatry, Florence, April 18–22, 2017.
26. Reeve J, Jang H. What teachers say and do to support students' autonomy during a learning activity. J Educ Psychol 2006;98(1):209–18.
27. Watkins CE. Listening, learning, and development in psychoanalytic supervision: A self psychology perspective. Psychoanal Psychol 2016;33(3):437–71.

28. Watkins CE. Self-psychology and psychoanalytic supervision: some thoughts on a contextualized perspective. Int J Psychoanal Self Psychol 2016;11(3):276–92.
29. Loo JL, Ang JK, Subhas N, et al. Learning psychodynamic psychiatry in Southeast Asia. Psychodyn Psychiatry 2017;45(1):45–57.
30. Woon LS, Kanapathy A, Zakaria H, et al. An integrative approach to treatment-resistant obsessive-compulsive disorder. Psychodyn Psychiatry 2017;45(2):237–57.
31. Javanbakht A, San'ati M. Psychiatry and psychoanalysis in Iran. J Am Acad Psychoanal Dyn Psychiatry 2006;34(3):405–14.
32. The World Psychiatric Association General Assembly Minutes. Berlin, October, 2017.

Where Is the Evidence for "Evidence-Based" Therapy?

Jonathan Shedler, PhD

KEYWORDS

• Evidence-based therapy • Empirically supported therapy • Psychotherapy • Psychotherapy outcome • Cognitive behavior therapy • CBT • Depression • Anxiety

KEY POINTS

- The term *evidence-based therapy* has become a de facto code word for manualized therapy—most often brief, highly scripted forms of cognitive behavior therapy.
- It is widely asserted that "evidence-based" therapies are scientifically proven and superior to other forms of psychotherapy. Empirical research does not support these claims.
- Empirical research shows that "evidence-based" therapies are weak treatments. Their benefits are trivial, few patients get well, and even the trivial benefits do not last.
- Troubling research practices paint a misleading picture of the actual benefits of "evidence-based" therapies, including sham control groups, cherry-picked patient samples, and suppression of negative findings.

Buzzword. noun. An important-sounding usually technical word or phrase often of little meaning used chiefly to impress.

"Evidence-based therapy" has become a marketing buzzword. The term "evidence based" comes from medicine. It gained attention in the 1990s and was initially a call for critical thinking. Proponents of evidence-based medicine recognized that "We've always done it this way" is poor justification for medical decisions. Medical decisions should integrate individual clinical expertise, patients' values and preferences, and relevant scientific research.[1]

But the term *evidence based* has come to mean something very different for psychotherapy. It has been appropriated to promote a specific ideology and agenda. It is now used as a code word for manualized therapy—most often brief, one-size-fits-all forms of cognitive behavior therapy (CBT). "Manualized" means the therapy is conducted by following an instruction manual. The treatments are often

Disclosure Statement: No conflicts to disclose.

 This article is adapted from Shedler J. Where is the evidence for "evidence-based" therapy? *Journal of Psychological Therapies in Primary Care* 2015;4:47–59. The material was originally presented as a keynote address at the Limbus Critical Psychotherapy Conference, Devon, England, November 1, 2014.

Department of Psychiatry, University of Colorado School of Medicine, Denver, CO 80045, USA
E-mail address: jonathan@shedler.com

Psychiatr Clin N Am 41 (2018) 319–329
https://doi.org/10.1016/j.psc.2018.02.001 psych.theclinics.com
0193-953X/18/

Abbreviations

CBT	cognitive behavior therapy
PTSD	posttraumatic stress disorder

standardized or scripted in ways that leave little room for addressing the needs of individual patients.

Behind the "evidence-based" therapy movement lies a master narrative that increasingly dominates the mental health landscape. The master narrative goes something like this: "In the dark ages, therapists practiced unproven, unscientific therapy. Evidence-based therapies are scientifically proven and superior." The narrative has become a justification for all-out attacks on traditional talk therapy—that is, therapy aimed at fostering self-examination and self-understanding in the context of an ongoing, meaningful therapy relationship.

Here is a small sample of what proponents of "evidence-based" therapy say in public: "The empirically supported psychotherapies are still not widely practiced. As a result, many patients *do not have access to adequate treatment*" (emphasis added).[2] Note the linguistic sleight-of-hand: If the therapy is not "evidence based" (read, manualized), it is inadequate. Other proponents of "evidence-based" therapies go further in denigrating relationship-based, insight-oriented therapy: "The disconnect between what clinicians do and what science has discovered is an unconscionable embarrassment."[3]

The news media promulgate the master narrative. The *Washington Post* ran an article titled "Is your therapist a little behind the times?" which likened traditional talk therapy to pre-scientific medicine when "healers commonly used ineffective and often injurious practices such as blistering, purging and bleeding." *Newsweek* sounded a similar note with an article titled, "Ignoring the evidence: Why do Psychologists reject science?"

Note how the language leads to a form of McCarthyism. Because proponents of brief, manualized therapies have appropriated the term "evidence-based," it has become nearly impossible to have an intelligent discussion about what constitutes good therapy. Anyone who questions "evidence-based" therapy risks being branded anti-evidence and anti-science.

One might assume, in light of the strong claims for "evidence-based" therapies and the public denigration of other therapies, that there must be extremely strong scientific evidence for their benefits. There is not. There is a yawning chasm between what we are told research shows and what research actually shows.

Empirical research actually shows that "evidence-based" therapies are ineffective for most patients most of the time. First, I discuss what empirical research really shows. I then take a closer look at troubling practices in "evidence-based" therapy research.

PART I: WHAT RESEARCH REALLY SHOWS

Research shows that "evidence-based" therapies are weak treatments. Their benefits are trivial. Most patients do not get well. Even the trivial benefits do not last.

This may be different from what you have been taught. It is incompatible with the master narrative. I will not ask you to accept my word for any of this. That is why I will discuss and quote primary sources.

In the Beginning

The gold standard of evidence in "evidence-based" therapy research is the randomized controlled trial. Patients with a specific psychiatric diagnosis are randomly assigned to treatment or control groups and the study compares the groups.

The mother of all randomized controlled trials for psychotherapy is the *National Institute of Mental Health (NIMH) Treatment of Depression Collaborative Research Program*. It was the first large-scale, multisite study of what are now called "evidence-based" therapies. The study included 3 active treatments: manualized CBT, manualized interpersonal therapy, and antidepressant medication. The control group got a placebo pill and clinical management but not psychotherapy. The study began in the mid-1970s and the first major findings were published in 1989.

For the last quarter of a century, we have been told that the NIMH study showed that CBT, interpersonal therapy, and antidepressant medication are "empirically validated" treatments for depression. We have been told that these treatments were proven effective. I focus here on CBT because the term *evidence-based therapy* most often refers to CBT and its variants.

The primary outcome measure in the NIMH study was the 54-point *Hamilton Depression Rating Scale*. The difference between the CBT treatment group and the placebo control group was 1.2 points.[4] The 1.2-point difference between the CBT and control group is trivial and clinically meaningless. It does not pass the "So what?" test. It does not pass the "Does it matter?" test. It does not pass the "Why should anyone care?" test.

How could there be such a mismatch between what we have been told versus what the study actually found? You may be wondering whether the original researchers did not present the data clearly. That is not the case. The first major research report from the NIMH study was published in 1989 in *Archives of General Psychiatry*.[4] The authors wrote: "There was limited evidence of the specific effectiveness of interpersonal psychotherapy and *none for cognitive behavior therapy*" (emphasis added). That is what the original research article reports.

In 1994, the principal investigator wrote a comprehensive review of what we learned from the study, titled "The NIMH Treatment of Depression Collaborative Research Program: Where we began and where we are."[5] Writing in careful academic language, the principal investigator stated, "What is most striking in the follow-up findings is the relatively small percentage of patients who remain in treatment, fully recover, and remain completely well throughout the 18-month follow-up period." The percentage is so small that it "raises questions about whether the potency of the short-term treatments for depression has been oversold."[5]

What was that percentage, actually? It turns out that only 24% of the patients got well and stayed well. In other words, about 75%—the overwhelming majority—did not get well. How can this be? We have been told the opposite for one-quarter of a century. We have been told that manualized CBT is powerful and effective.

Statistically Significant Does Not Mean Effective

The word *significant* gives rise to considerable misunderstanding. In the English language, *significant* is a synonym for important or meaningful. In statistics, *significant* is a term of art with a technical definition, pertaining to the probability of an observed finding.[a] "Statistically significant" does not indicate that findings are of scientific import (a point emphasized in a recent statement by the American Statistical Association[6]). They absolutely do not mean that patients get well or even that they improve in any clinically meaningfully way.

[a] More precisely, "the probability under a specified statistical model that a statistical summary of the data (eg, the sample mean difference between two compared groups) would be equal to or more extreme than its observed value."[6]

There is a mismatch between the questions studies of "evidence-based" therapy tend to ask versus what patients, clinicians, and health care policymakers need to know. Studies are conducted by academic researchers who often have little or no clinical practice experience, who may not appreciate the challenges and complexities therapists and patients face in real-world practice. Writing in *American Psychologist*, eminent CBT researcher Alan Kazdin noted, "Researchers often *do not know* if clients receiving an evidence-based treatment have improved in everyday life or changed in a way that makes a difference" (emphasis added).[7]

Major misunderstandings arise when researchers "disseminate" research findings to patients, policymakers, and practitioners. Researchers speak of "significant" treatment benefits, referring to statistical significance. Most people understandably but mistakenly take this to mean that patients get well or at least meaningfully better.

Few other disciplines emphasize "significance" instead of actual change. When there is a meaningful treatment benefit, investigators emphasize that, not "significance." If a drug is effective in lowering blood pressure, we report how much it lowers blood pressure. If we have an effective weight loss program, we report that the average person in the program lost 20 pounds, or 30 pounds, or whatever. If we have a drug that lowers cholesterol, we report how much it lowers cholesterol. We would not focus on statistical significance. When researchers focus on statistical significance, something is being hidden.

I am embarrassed that when I first wrote about the NIMH depression study, I assumed that the 1.2-point difference between the CBT group and the placebo control group was statistically significant, even if clinically irrelevant.[8] I assumed this was why the study was widely cited as scientific evidence for CBT. When I subsequently examined the primary sources more closely, I discovered that the 1.2-point difference on the depression rating scale was not *even* statistically significant. It was difficult to wrap my head around the notion that widespread claims that the study provided scientific support for CBT had no basis in the actual data. This seems to be a case where the master narrative trumped the facts.

Research Continues, Treatment Benefits Do Not

The NIMH findings were published more than 25 years ago. Surely, research findings for CBT must have improved over time. Let's jump ahead to the most recent state-of-the-art randomized controlled trial for depression.[9] The study included 341 depressed patients randomly assigned to 16 sessions of manualized CBT or 16 sessions of manualized psychodynamic therapy. The 2 treatments did not differ in effectiveness. The study was published in 2013 in the *American Journal of Psychiatry*. The authors wrote, "One notable finding was that only 22.7% of the patients achieved remission."[9] They continued, "Our findings indicate that a substantial proportion of patients . . . require more than time-limited therapy to achieve remission." In other words, about 75% of patients did not get well. It is essentially the same finding reported in the NIMH study one-quarter of a century earlier.

The appropriate conclusion to be drawn from both of these major studies is that brief manualized therapies are ineffective for most depressed patients most of the time.

I have described the earliest major study and the most recent. What about the research in between? The findings are largely the same. The research is summarized in a review paper in *Psychological Bulletin* by Drew Westen and colleagues.[10] The paper is a detailed, comprehensive literature review of manualized CBT for depression and anxiety disorders.

The researchers found that the average patient who received manualized CBT for depression remained clinically depressed after treatment, with an average *Beck Depression Inventory* score greater than 10. What about conditions besides depression? How about panic disorder? Panic seems to be the condition for which brief, manualized CBT work best. However, the average patient who received "evidence-based" treatment for panic disorder still had panic attacks almost weekly and still endorsed 4 of 7 symptoms listed in the *Diagnostic and Statistical Manual of Mental Disorders*, 4th edition. These patients did not get well either.

Another finding was that the benefits of manualized "evidence-based" therapies are temporary. Treatment outcome is typically measured the day treatment ends. But when patients are followed over time, treatment benefits evaporate. The majority of patients who receive an "evidence-based" therapy—more than 50%—seek treatment again within 6 to 12 months for the same condition. This finding should give investigators pause. It would also be a mistake to conclude that those who do not seek additional treatment are well. Some may have gotten well. Many may have simply given up on psychotherapy.

Even ardent CBT advocates have acknowledged that manualized CBT offers lasting help to few. Writing in *Psychological Science in the Public Interest*, eminent CBT researcher Steven Hollon noted "Only about half of all patients respond to any given intervention, and only about a third eventually meet the criteria for remission. . . . Moreover, most patients will not stay well once they get better unless they receive ongoing treatment."[2] Ironically, this was written by the same researcher who declared other forms of psychotherapy "inadequate." Sadly, such information reaches few clinicians and fewer patients. I wonder what the public and policy makes would think if they knew these are the same treatments described publicly as "evidence-based," "scientifically proven," and "the gold standard."

PART 2: A CLOSER LOOK AT RESEARCH PRACTICES

In this section, I address some research practices behind the claims for manualized, "evidence-based" therapies. I address the following issues: First, most patients are never counted. Second, the control groups are shams. Third, manualized, "evidence-based" therapy has not shown superiority to any other form of psychotherapy. Fourth, data are being hidden.

Most Patients Are Never Counted

In the typical randomized controlled trial for "evidence-based" therapies, about two-thirds of the patients are excluded from the studies a priori.[10] Sometimes exclusion rates exceed 80%. That is, the patients have the diagnosis and seek treatment, but because of the study's inclusion and exclusion criteria, they are excluded from participation. The higher the exclusion rates, the better the outcomes.[11] Typically, the patients who are excluded are those who meet criteria for more than one psychiatric diagnosis, or have personality pathology, or are considered unstable, or who may be suicidal. In other words, they are the patients we treat in real-world practice. The patients included in the research studies are not representative of any real-world clinical population.

Here is some simple arithmetic. Approximately two-thirds of patients who seek treatment are excluded from the research studies. Of the one-third who are treated, about one-half show improvement. This is about 16% of the patients who initially presented for treatment. But this is just patients who show "improvement." If we consider patients who actually get well, we are down to about 11% of those who originally sought treatment. If we consider patients who get well and stay well, we are down to 5% or fewer. In other words, scientific research demonstrates that "evidence-based" treatments are effective and have lasting benefits for approximately 5% of the patients who seek treatment. Here is another way to look at it (**Fig. 1**). The iceberg represents the patients who seek treatment for a psychiatric condition—depression, generalized anxiety, and so on. The tip of the iceberg represents the patients described in the "evidence-based" therapy research literature. All the rest—the huge part of the iceberg below the water—do not get counted. The research methods render them invisible.

Control Groups Are Shams

Second point: The control group is usually a sham. What do I mean? I mean that "evidence-based" therapies are almost never compared to legitimate alternative therapies. The control group is usually a foil invented by researchers committed to demonstrating the benefits of CBT. In other words, the control group is a fake treatment that is intended to fail.

A state-of-the-art, NIMH-funded study of posttraumatic stress disorder (PTSD) provides a good illustration of a sham control group.[12] The study focused on "single incident" PTSD. The patients were previously healthy. They developed PTSD after experiencing a specific identifiable trauma. The study claims to compare psychodynamic therapy with a form of CBT called prolonged exposure therapy. It claims to show that CBT is superior to psychodynamic therapy. This is what it says in the discussion section: "[CBT] was superior to [psychodynamic therapy] in decreasing

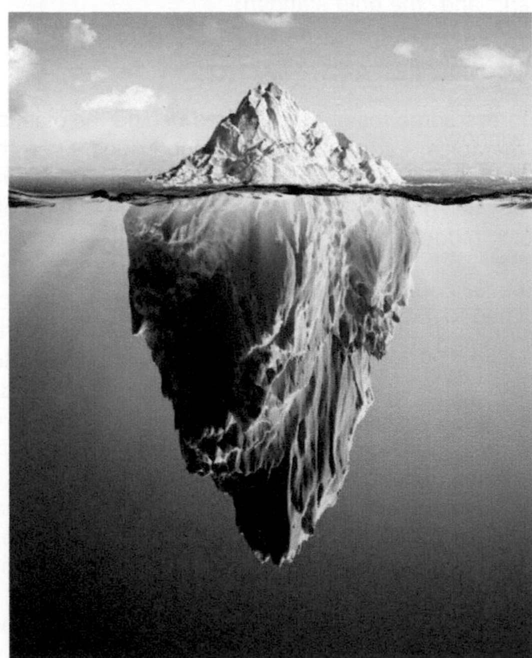

Fig. 1. Most patients are never counted. (*Courtesy of* iStock by Getty Images, St. Louis, Missouri.)

symptoms of PTSD and depression, enhancing functioning . . . and increasing overall improvement."

That is what was communicated to the media, the public, and policymakers. If you read the fine print and do a little homework, things look very different. Who were the therapists who provided the "psychodynamic" treatment? Were they experienced, qualified, psychodynamic therapists? No. It turns out that they were graduate students. They received 2 days of training in psychodynamic therapy from another graduate student—a graduate student in a research laboratory committed to CBT. In contrast, the therapists who provided CBT received 5 days of training by the developer of the treatment, world-famous author and researcher Edna Foa. That is not exactly a level playing field.

But that was the least of the problems. The so-called psychodynamic therapists were prohibited from discussing the trauma that brought the patient to treatment. Imagine that—you seek treatment for PTSD because you have experienced a traumatic event, and your therapist refuses to discuss it. The therapists were trained to change the topic when patients brought up their traumatic experiences.

If a clinician practiced this way in the real world, it could be considered malpractice. In "evidence-based" therapy research, that is considered a control group, and a basis for claims that CBT is superior to psychodynamic therapy.[b] Even with the sham therapy control condition, the advantage of CBT still disappeared at long-term follow up—but you would have to sift through the results section with a fine-toothed comb to know this.

The "Superiority" of Evidence-Based Therapy Is a Myth

In case you are thinking the PTSD study is unusual—perhaps cherry-picked to make a point—that is not the case. There is a comprehensive review of the psychotherapy research literature that addresses this very question.[15] It focused on randomized controlled trials for both anxiety and depression. The researchers examined studies that claimed to compare an "evidence-based" therapy with an alternative form of psychotherapy. The researchers examined more than 2500 abstracts. After closer examination, they winnowed that down to 149 studies that looked like they might actually compare an "evidence-based" therapy with another legitimate form of therapy. But when they finished, there were only 14 studies that compared "evidence-based" therapy with a control group that received anything resembling bona fide psychotherapy. These studies showed no advantages whatever for "evidence-based" therapies.

Many studies claimed to use control groups that received "treatment as usual." But "treatment as usual" turned out to be "predominantly 'treatments' that *did not include any psychotherapy.*"[15] I am not interpreting or paraphrasing. This is a quotation from the original article. In other words, "evidence-based" therapies were not compared with other forms of legitimate psychotherapy. They were compared and found "superior" to doing nothing. Alternatively, they were compared with control groups that received sham psychotherapy where therapists had their hands tied—as in the PTSD study described above.

This literature review was published in a conservative scholarly journal and the authors stated their conclusions in careful academic language. They concluded, "Currently, there is insufficient evidence to suggest that transporting an evidence-

[b] Shockingly, when a letter to the editor called the researchers on the fact that the sham therapy control condition was not psychodynamic therapy, they doubled down and insisted it was.[13,14]

based therapy to routine care that already involves psychotherapy will improve the quality of services." In somewhat plainer English, "evidence-based" therapies are not more effective than any other form of psychotherapy. That is what the scientific literature actually shows. That is not just my opinion. It is the official scientific policy conclusion of the American Psychological Association.[16]

Data Are Suppressed

"Publication bias" is a well-known phenomenon in research. Publication bias refers to the fact that studies with positive results—those that show the outcomes desired by the investigators—tend to get published. Studies that fail to show the desired outcome tend not to get published. For this reason, published research can provide a biased or skewed picture of actual research findings. There is a name for this phenomenon, it is called the "file-drawer effect." For every published study with positive results, how many studies with negative results are hidden in researchers' file drawers? How can you prove there are file drawers stuffed with negative results? It turns out there is a way to do this. There are statistical methods to estimate how many unpublished studies have negative results that are hidden from view.

A team of researchers tackled this question for research on CBT for depression.[17] They found that the published benefits of CBT are exaggerated by 75% owing to publication bias. How do you find out something like this? How can you know what is hidden in file drawers? You know by examining what is called a funnel plot. The idea is actually quite simple. Suppose you are conducting a poll—"Are US citizens for or against building a border wall with Mexico?"—and you examine very small samples of only 3 people. The results can be all over the place. Depending on the 3 people you happen to select, it may look like 100% of citizens favor a wall or 100% oppose it. With small sample sizes, you see a wide scatter or range of results. As sample sizes get larger, the findings stabilize and converge.

If you graph the findings—in this case, the relationship between sample size and treatment benefit—you get a plot that looks like a funnel (**Fig. 2**, left). Studies with smaller sample sizes show more variability in results, and studies with larger sample sizes tend to converge on more similar values. That is what it should look like if data are not being hidden. In fact, what it looks like is something like the graph on

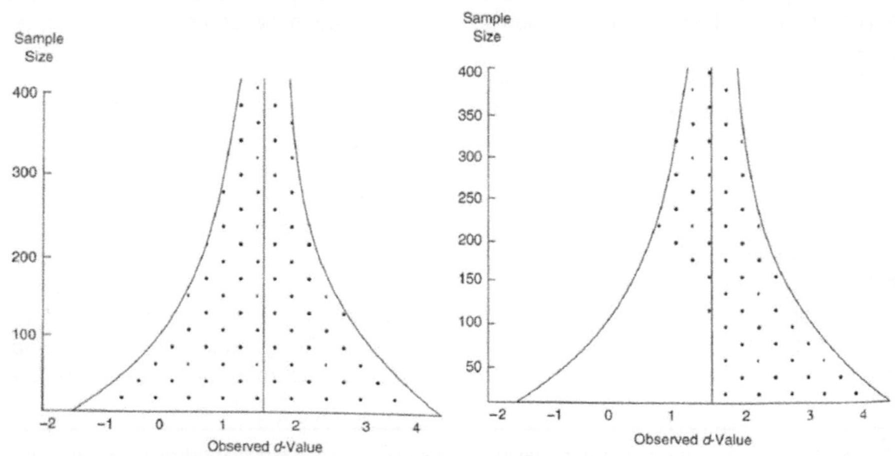

Fig. 2. Sample funnel plot. (*Courtesy of* J. Shedler, PhD, Denver, CO.)

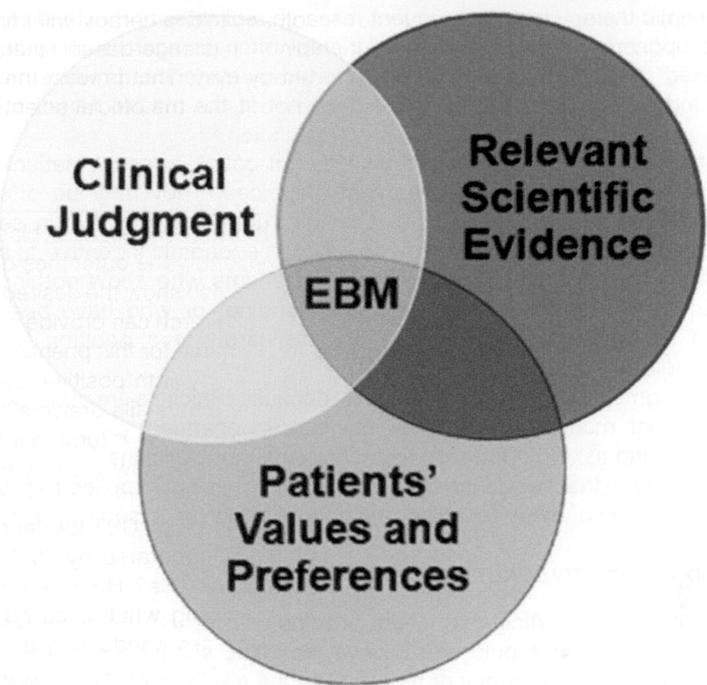

Fig. 3. What is evidence-based medicine (EBM)? (*From* Sackett DL, Rosenberg WM, Gray JA, et al. Evidence based medicine: what it is and what it isn't. BMJ 1996;312(7023):71–2; with permission.)

the right (see **Fig. 2**). The data points that are supposed to be in the lower left area of the graph are missing.[c]

WHAT "EVIDENCE-BASED" IS SUPPOSED TO MEAN?

What is "evidence-based" supposed to mean? I noted earlier that the term originated in medicine. Evidence-based medicine was meant to be the integration of:

a. Relevant scientific evidence,
b. Patients' values and preferences, and
c. The individual experience and clinical judgment of practitioners (**Fig. 3**)[1,19]

What has happened to these ideas in psychotherapy? "Relevant scientific evidence" no longer counts, because proponents of "evidence-based" therapies ignore evidence for therapies that are not manualized and scripted. In 2010, I published an article in *American Psychologist* titled, "The Efficacy of Psychodynamic Psychotherapy."[20] The article demonstrates that the benefits of psychodynamic therapy are at least as large as those of therapies promoted as "evidence based"—and moreover, the benefits of

[c] There was public outcry when research revealed the extent of publication bias in clinical trials for antidepressant medication.[18] The bias was widely attributed to the influence of the pharmaceutical industry and conflicts of interest of investigators with financial ties to pharmaceutical companies. However, the publication bias for antidepressants medication pales in comparison with the publication bias for "evidence-based" therapy.

psychodynamic therapy last. Subsequent research replicates and extends these findings. Yet proponents of "evidence-based" therapy often disregard such evidence. "Evidence based" does not actually mean supported by evidence, it means manualized, scripted, and not psychodynamic. What does not fit the master narrative does not count.

"Patients' values and preferences" also do not count, because patients are not adequately informed or offered meaningful choices. They may be offered only brief manualized treatment and told it is the "gold standard." This serves the financial interests of health insurers, who have an economic incentive to shunt patients to the briefest, cheapest treatments.[21] Patients who know nothing of therapy aimed at self-reflection and self-understanding, or who have heard it only denigrated as inadequate or unscientific, are hardly in a position to exercise informed choice.

"Clinical judgment" also no longer matters, because clinicians are often expected to follow treatment manuals rather than exercise independent judgment. They are increasingly being asked to function as technicians, not clinicians.[d]

One could argue that "evidence based," as the term is now applied to psychotherapy, is a perversion of every founding principle of evidence-based medicine.

FACTS AND ALTERNATIVE FACTS

The information in this article may seem at odds with virtually all other respectable scholarly sources. Why should you believe me? You should not believe me. You should not take my word for any of this—or anyone else's word. I will leave you with 3 simple things to do to help sift truth from hyperbole. When somebody makes a claim for a treatment, any treatment, follow these 3 steps:

- Step 1: Say, "Show me the study." Ask for a reference, a citation, a PDF. Have the study put in your hands. Sometimes it does not exist.
- Step 2: If the study does exist, read it—especially the fine print.
- Step 3: Draw your own conclusions. Ask yourself: Do the actual methods and findings of the study justify the claim I heard?

If you make a practice of following these simple steps, you may make some shocking discoveries.

REFERENCES

1. Sackett DL, Rosenberg WM, Gray JA, et al. Evidence based medicine: what it is and what it isn't. BMJ 1996;312(7023):71–2.
2. Hollon SD, Thase ME, Markowitz JC. Treatment and prevention of depression. Psychol Sci Public Interest 2002;3(2):39–77.
3. Mischel W. Connecting clinical practice to scientific progress. Psychol Sci Public Interest 2008;9(2):i–ii.

---

[d] Lest the reader think this a misrepresentation or caricature, consider that prominent proponents of manualized therapy advocate treatment by minimally trained paraprofessionals. The journal *Psychological Science in the Public Interest*, the house organ of the Association for Psychological Science, published the following: "Many of these [evidence-based] interventions can be disseminated without highly trained and expensive personnel. . . . CBT is effective even when delivered by nondoctoral therapists or by health educators with little or no prior experience with CBT who received only a modest level of training . . . manuals and workbooks are available on user-friendly websites."[22] The devaluation of clinical expertise inherent in these statements requires no interpretation.

4. Elkin I, Shea MT, Watkins JT, et al. National Institute of Mental Health Treatment of Depression Collaborative Research Program. General effectiveness of treatments. Arch Gen Psychiatry 1989;46(11):971–82 [discussion: 983].
5. Elkin I. Treatment of depression collaborative research program: where we began and where we are. In: Bergin A, Garfield S, editors. Handbook of psychotherapy and behavior change. 4th edition. New York: Wiley; 1994. p. 114–39.
6. Wasserstein RL, Lazar NA. The ASA's statement on p-values: context, process, and purpose. Am Stat 2016;70:129–33. Available at: https://www.tandfonline.com/doi/full/10.1080/00031305.2016.1154108.
7. Kazdin AE. Arbitrary metrics: implications for identifying evidence-based treatments. Am Psychol 2006;61(1):42–9 [discussion: 62–71].
8. Shedler J. Where is the evidence for "evidence-based" therapy? Journal of Psychological Therapies in Primary Care 2015;4:47–59.
9. Driessen E, Van HL, Don FJ, et al. The efficacy of cognitive-behavioral therapy and psychodynamic therapy in the outpatient treatment of major depression: a randomized clinical trial. Am J Psychiatry 2013;170(9):1041–50.
10. Westen D, Novotny CM, Thompson-Brenner H. The empirical status of empirically supported psychotherapies: assumptions, findings, and reporting in controlled clinical trials. Psychol Bull 2004;130(4):631–63.
11. Westen D, Morrison K. A multidimensional meta-analysis of treatments for depression, panic, and generalized anxiety disorder: an empirical examination of the status of empirically supported therapies. J Consult Clin Psychol 2001; 69(6):875–99.
12. Gilboa-Schechtman E, Foa EB, Shafran N, et al. Prolonged exposure versus dynamic therapy for adolescent PTSD: a pilot randomized controlled trial. J Am Acad Child Adolesc Psychiatry 2010;49(10):1034–42.
13. Gilboa-Schechtman E, Shafran N, Foa EB, et al. Journal of the American Academy of Child & Adolescent Psychiatry 2011;50(5):522–4.
14. Wittmann L, Halpern J, Adams CB, et al. Prolonged exposure and psychodynamic treatment for posttraumatic stress disorder. J Am Acad Child Adolesc Psychiatry 2011;50(5):521–2 [author reply: 522–1].
15. Wampold BE, Budge SL, Laska KM, et al. Evidence-based treatments for depression and anxiety versus treatment-as-usual: a meta-analysis of direct comparisons. Clin Psychol Rev 2011;31(8):1304–12.
16. American Psychological Association. Recognition of psychotherapy effectiveness: the APA resolution. Psychotherapy 2013;50(1):98–101.
17. Cuijpers P, Smit F, Bohlmeijer E, et al. Efficacy of cognitive-behavioural therapy and other psychological treatments for adult depression: meta-analytic study of publication bias. Br J Psychiatry 2010;196(3):173–8.
18. Turner EH, Matthews AM, Linardatos E, et al. Selective publication of antidepressant trials and its influence on apparent efficacy. N Engl J Med 2008;358(3):252–60.
19. APA Presidential Task Force on Evidence-Based Practice. Evidence-based practice in psychology. Am Psychol 2006;61(4):271–85.
20. Shedler J. The efficacy of psychodynamic psychotherapy. Am Psychol 2010; 65(2):98–109.
21. Bendat M. In name only? Mental health parity or illusory reform. Psychodyn Psychiatry 2014;42(3):353–75
22. Baker TB, McFall RM, Shoham V. Current status and future prospects of clinical psychology: toward a scientifically principled approach to mental and behavioral health care. Psychol Sci Public Interest 2008;9(2):67–103.

Engineering Neurobiological Systems: Addiction

Brian Johnson, MD[a,b]

KEYWORDS

• Addiction • Biological engineering • Neuropsychoanalysis • SEEKING • Opioid • Tobacco

KEY POINTS

- Psychodynamic treatment of addiction must take into account that there is an addictive drug industry, both legal and illicit, and that huge profits are made by injuring and killing people. This fact propitiates the therapeutic alliance between patient and analyst and minimizes countertransference stigma and frustration.
- Psychodynamic treatment of addiction requires an understanding of drug effects on the brain. Neuropsychoanalysis involves correlation of psychoanalytic psychology and clinical patient experiences with neurobiology and therefore fulfills this requirement.
- Engineering models are based on neurobiology. Models facilitate efficacy of treatment.
- A drug cannot be addictive unless it can change the ventral tegmental dopaminergic SEEKING system, resulting in changed thinking by the drug user. This change is best described as "mind control," meaning the drug user brings the drug seller money despite the user's knowledge of being injured and possibly killed by the drug.
- The SEEKING system is the neurobiological correlate of the will, the experience of drive operating within us. Knowledge that the will of the patient has been taken over by a drug dealer is required of the psychodynamic treater and must be interpreted to the patient.

INTRODUCTION

One hundred million people were killed by tobacco in the 20th century, and we are on track for 1 billion killed in the 21st century.[1] The chance of someone using illicit drugs is 80 times higher if they start inhaling cigarettes before the age of 15.[2] Given that the average age of onset of smoking is 13,[3] most victims are captured as children. Alcohol, the other addictive drug legal when the United States was founded in

---

Disclosure Statement: The authors have no financial arrangements or affiliations with any commercial entities whose products, research, or services are discussed in this report.
[a] Boston Psychoanalytic Society, Newton Centre, MA, USA; [b] Department of Psychiatry, State University of New York (SUNY) Upstate Medical University, 750 East Adams Street, Syracuse, NY 13210, USA
E-mail address: johnsonb@upstate.edu

Psychiatr Clin N Am 41 (2018) 331–339
https://doi.org/10.1016/j.psc.2018.01.011 **psych.theclinics.com**
0193-953X/18/

1789, kills 4% of the population.[4] Twenty-five percent of Americans die from using drugs (**Table 1**). Selling addictive drugs in the United States generates $845 billion per year, 5% of the gross domestic product (**Table 2**).

We know this, but not consciously. We act as if we have not noticed. The size of the mass killing is an order of magnitude greater than the holocaust or Stalin's murders. It is going on right now. The wish not to know is powerful. Words, the polar opposite of unconsciously driven destructive behaviors, are our solution. The psychoanalytic enterprise is to help make our patients and our society conscious.

The definition of addiction is, "Repeated use despite harm." If one inhales sticks of dirt, carcinogens, and nicotine, every stick creates harm. Social cigarette use is rare. Alcohol is more variable. One can drink every day and live to an old age. Alcohol and marijuana are drugs that usually affect people adversely when they start using in the morning. Most users do not become addicted. One of the problems about understanding drug addiction is that one cannot simply project one's own experience into another. The effect of drugs with addictive potential depends on the character of the person using the drug. Character function is complex and includes genetic predispositions. But genes are designed to undergo epigenetic changes, as humans develop in a social surround. We could say as an approximation that we are going to use psychoanalytic models to simplify the complexity of behaviors that have contributions from biological, psychological, and social sources.[5] However, in addiction, the neurobiology of addictive behaviors is so important that it is more accurate to call them engineering models.

ENGINEERING MODELS

"The purpose of an abstraction hierarchy is to hide information and manage complexity. To be useful, biological engineering abstraction hierarchies must allow individuals to work at any one level of complexity without regard for the details that define other levels, yet allow for the principled exchange of limited information across levels."[16] As defined by the International Council on Systems Engineering, "A system is a construct or collection of different elements that together produce results not obtainable by the elements alone."[17] Here we combine elements of neurobiology, psychoanalytic psychology, and the grim reality of the addictive drug industry and its victims, to construct a systems engineering approach to treatment and research.

Neurobiological concepts are used here to build engineering models. Arguments over whether every aspect of the model is correct are not important. Engineers

Table 1
Drugs kill one-fourth of Americans

Drug	American Deaths/Year
Tobacco	480,000
Alcohol	88,000
Opioid overdose	59,000
Benzodiazepine overdose	9000
Cocaine	6784
Methamphetamine	5740
Total deaths from drugs	648,524
Total deaths in United States	2,626,418

Data from Refs.[6–8]

Table 2 Income of addictive drug industry: $845 billion, 5% US gross domestic product	
Industry	**Sales ($ Billions)**
Benzodiazepine	509
Alcohol	212
Tobacco	50
Marijuana—if legalized in the United States	45
Mexican/Columbian drug cartels	29
Opioid medications	19
Comparison—US auto	70

Data from Refs.[9–15]

want to make things happen in the real world. Addicted patients may die. We want engineering models that help them stay alive. Although the neuropsychoanalytic Addiction Medicine Service at the State University of New York uses at least 11 engineering models as a basis of making interpretations, this brief work considers a central model about drive and instinct to illustrate how the approach is used. A longer exposition about neuropsychoanalysis can be found in a work by Johnson and Mosri.[18]

THE SEEKING SYSTEM AND ITS INSTINCTUAL SUBORDINATES

Panksepp[19,20] used animal/brain pathway research to improve our ability to understand a notable confusion in Freud's thinking: the difference between drive and instinct. In neuropsychoanalysis, the psychoanalytic concept of drive is correlated with SEEKING,[18] a dopaminergic pathway that runs from the ventral tegmental area at the top of the midbrain along the basal forebrain; through the hypothalamus where it is tuned by inputs about food, water, and sex; and synapses with the nucleus accumbens. From this point, branches go to brain areas involved in motivated behaviors. Dopamine pathways are distinctly frontal and ventral—brain regions that are connected with motor function—in contrast with other neurotransmitters like norepinephrine or serotonin that stimulate the brain generally including all 4 cortical lobes and dorsal as well as ventral subcortical areas.

Plants don't need brains because they grow wherever a seed lands. Animals need a source of motivation to move through their environment to find the resources to stay alive and procreate. The particular goal of SEEKING shifts according to hypothalamic input. If the hypothalamus detects dehydration, the animal SEEKS water. If the animal drinks and then needs sex, the goal is shifted. There is no need for consciousness; this is a midbrain function. Consciousness tends to be awakened by the frustration of unpleasure,[21] of not automatically getting what is desired. Looking ahead to addiction, inhaling 20 cigarettes per day is not particularly conscious. It is only when in an environment in which the next cigarette is difficult to use that the addicted individual begins to think consciously about what to do to be able to inhale nicotine.

Although the SEEKING pathway constantly goads animals like us into investigating our environment, an activity that is pleasant in its own right, we have 6 instinctual (not drive) systems with identified neural pathways. CARE, LUST and PLAY are also pleasant. The CARE system of mammals is built on the LUST system present in many animals. Turtles lust after each other, creating fertilized eggs. The babies hatch and are on their own from birth. Mammals instinctually CARE for their children. They are just so darned cute! This feeling requires hormonal input to be experienced.[22] If you are the older sibling of a newborn, you may have no feelings that this baby is cute. You are more likely to have RAGE turned on than CARE. Feelings about children change at puberty when hormones modulate both LUST and CARE systems.[22] PLAY is built into mammals to rehearse adult activities in a safe way. Children want to wrestle each other and their parents, rehearsing closeness without damage, rehearsing fighting, rehearsing competition. It feels good.

The pleasure principle is defined as a principle governing human psychological functioning, whereby unpleasure motivates psychological and behavioral activity.[21] We hate not to have what we want when we want it. We are happy to have pleasure but don't have it compulsively. We hate unpleasure and do everything we can to disengage from it. The next 3 systems generate unpleasure.

At the healthiest end of human relatedness, when someone impinges on us in a way that makes us angry (RAGE), we either move away from that person or if possible or talk through what they did that made us unhappy so that it doesn't happen again. Many people, especially children, feel trapped in human environments where RAGE is turned on constantly by interpersonal attacks. There is no talking things through. RAGE is complicated by a demoralizing sense of helplessness.

FEAR does not necessarily have anything to do with interpersonal relatedness. It is a signal that tissue damage may ensue. One can have this feeling when one gets near a cliff. Unfortunately, one can have it in one's own family. One of our patients was 11 when her father appeared to be beating his girlfriend to death. The father told her if she called the police, he would kill her too. The police were called by a neighbor, the girlfriend asked for a final kiss on her bloody, beaten face, believing that she would die. This kiss of the bloody, beaten face became a flashbulb memory. The patient developed posttraumatic stress disorder. When she got to work in the morning she was always careful to watch that another employee went in first, "In case a man was in the building who might kill me." Years later this patient experienced the "high" of alcoholic drinking as turning off the constant signal of fear that she might be killed any time.

PANIC is turned on by separation. Being with others feels great because of stimulation of the endogenous opioid system. Losing someone hurts. Panksepp explained that the PANIC system is built into animals so that they stay safely with others of their band.[20] It is evident in work with addicted patients that many people experience being completely alone, even in their family.

RAGE, FEAR, and PANIC are turned on in families in which parents behave badly, a common phenomenon. An epidemiologic study found that 25% of Americans meet the adult criteria for antisocial personality: 32% of men, 18% of women.[23] Behavioral manifestations include repeatedly performing acts that are grounds for arrest, conning others, aggressiveness as indicated by repeated physical fights, reckless disregard for the safety of self and others, repeated failure to sustain consistent work behavior or honor financial obligations, and lack of remorse: being indifferent to or rationalizing having hurt, mistreated, or stolen from another.

It hurts to be with people who are not emotionally available. New York University psychoanalyst Anne Erreich defined unconscious fantasy[24] as "a subset of the domain of mental representations, those concerned with conflicting wishes, affects, and defensive maneuvers." In a description of the function of unconscious fantasy, Erreich wrote[24]:

> *Avoidantly attached children have had innumerable experiences of having their neediness rejected by their mother, and so, despite signs of physiologic distress, they rebuff or ignore their mother when frightened, denying their neediness and/or*

doing to their mothers what has been done to them. Especially given what is known about the sophisticated cognitive abilities of even very young infants, it is hard to imagine an infant or toddler who doesn't initially register consciously its mother's rebuff. More likely the early accumulation of this type of experience turns initial awareness into an out-of-awareness prediction or expectation, resulting in a defensive inhibition of the subjective awareness of neediness, as well as need-seeking behavior. This dynamic eventually evolves into a characterological style of relating to self and others. As Paley (2007) puts it, "Since predictions incorporate past experience and learning, the past biases current experience. In a sense we learn to predict what to expect from the future and then live the future that we expect."

The unconscious fantasy of many addicted patients is that persons one depends on ignore one's need for closeness. This expectation is applied to current relationships. Even the most attentive psychodynamic clinician may not meet the needs of the avoidantly attached patient. For these patients, closeness constantly hurts. The relationship causes intolerable unpleasure.

The instinctual systems RAGE, FEAR, and PANIC are awful to experience. In families in which children are enjoyed and engaged, childhood is excellent. In families in which unpleasant feelings are constant and inescapable, teenagers look for drugs that turn off misery. Adolescents are the hardest addicted population to engage because they have just learned how to suffer less. They idealize their drug experience. They do all they can to escape treatment that they experience as having the potential to turn pain back on.

Another engineering model is fully developed in a report called Addiction and Will.[25] Adolescent drug use changes the SEEKING system. The psychology of the person reorients to accommodate the brain change. This is the denial system of addiction. If one listens carefully to patients who are explaining why they use drugs, the explanation actually makes no sense to an outsider. The explanation for drug use explains to the addicted person alone why they are using a drug that they know causes harm. For example, when asking someone why they inhale burning tobacco, a 50% mortality rate drug, one gets explanations such as, "We all have to die sometime," or "I need something to do with my hands," or "It relieves stress." The will of the addicted person has been taken over by the drug seller. The addicted person is not conscious that this has happened. Their experience is that they are the ones who want to use the drug. The reality is that by virtue of using a drug that changes the SEEKING system, other aspects of brain function shift to protect the false fitness signal as if the drug is necessary for life.[26]

Thus the sellers of addictive drugs have a product that controls the mind of the drug user. One notices, for example, that children frequently go from finding cigarettes aversive and begging their parents to stop, to urgently wanting cigarettes a few years later after beginning to use them. Now the SEEKING pathway demands food, water, sex, and nicotine. This neurobiologic change is the key to the finances of the addictive drug industry. If the drug seller can market the drug well enough to get people to take the drug into their brain, there is a brain change. The addicted person now has something that originated from outside them but has become permanently lodged within them. Abstinence despite constant SEEKING-mediated urges to use the drug again is the only way to escape further damage. No wonder step one of Alcoholics Anonymous starts with, "We admitted that we were powerless over alcohol." No wonder some people go to Alcoholics Anonymous for decades after becoming sober! Returning to use of tobacco or alcohol after falling under the influence of the sellers of the drug by virtue of a permanent brain change returns control of the person to the seller of the drug. This is the mind control nature of addictive drugs. One is powerless over drug use.

Many conventional drug treatments involve supplying the type of drug that the patients are addicted to with little attention to character. For example, methadone maintenance involves staff that inspect each patient before dosing to look for signs of intoxication, high-tech systems pour the methadone dose, nurses observe drug ingestion. The whole treatment is oriented around supplying a drug in the opioid class and monitoring safe use. Outcomes at 4.5 years indicate more than a 1% annual mortality rate, 32% opioid-positive urine drug screens, and 4 days of heroin use over the last month.[27] This is the harm reduction approach to addiction treatment.

The alternative partially described here poses substantial challenges to the psychodynamic clinician. The patient is using drugs that threaten their life. Character issues that evolved during childhood make drug use appealing as a temporary solution to feelings that are experienced as intolerable. Psychological trauma is ubiquitous. Change in character structure is needed so that the automatic solution of drug use to stifle feelings is shifted to something safer and more long lasting as a solution. Outcomes for this type of treatment are unknown. Research support is needed to establish what happens to addicted persons who engage in patient-centered psychodynamic treatments that follow the lead of the patient's associations and dreams to address character issues and other fundamental disorders underlying addiction rather than instructional or medication-oriented treatments in which the help provided is determined by the philosophy of the treaters and applied to all patients in the same way.

How people get recruited to addictive drug use:

- They can't stand the constant trauma of RAGE, FEAR, and PANIC. They use drugs to turn the signal off. This form of addiction can be ameliorated by helping the patient deal with their repressed trauma via psychoanalytic therapy. The trauma is remembered, understood, and worked through, and the need to use drugs addictively goes away. This is called *psychological addiction*.[28,29]
- Repeated use of addictive drugs changes the SEEKING system. Noxious drugs become urgently wanted. This is called *physical addiction*. Physical addiction is forever. An Alcoholics Anonymous aphorism that describes this is, "You can't change a pickle back into a cucumber."

We might return at the end of this brief exposition about drug addiction to ask the question, "What is the difference between a psychoanalytic model and an engineering neurobiology model?" The answer has implications for both treatment and research. Although psychoanalytic models may mention biology, it is never clear how the biology fits in. The models are based on clinical interactions. They are psychological models. "I saw a patient. They used free association. This is what I understand to be a model to use in the treatment, and to communicate what I do to other psychodynamic clinicians."

Engineering neurobiology models use dual aspect monism.[30] This means there is a correlation between the neurobiology and the clinical interaction. Using the example above, that someone says, "I am smoking cigarettes because I need something to do with my hands." The patient is not asked, "What comes to mind about doing something with your hands?" Instead there may be a statement from the treater, "This is a sign that your brain has been taken over by the tobacco company. Your explanation makes sense only inside you. All you are doing is restating, 'I urgently want cigarettes.'" This is a specific situation in which a model built on psychology alone would render patient and treater helpless to address a potentially fatal addiction.

In terms of research, engineering neurobiology models give an alternative to using purely psychological concepts such as the reward pathway. We can see that there is nothing rewarding about drug use. The concept of reward is also a purely psychological construct based on animal observations that specifically left out the brain and simply counted conditioned responses to conditioned stimuli.[19(p12)] By using the combination of a psychological concept of unconscious fantasy along with the neurobiology of the SEEKING system, a neuropsychoanalytic approach, we can begin to think about how trauma, the human penchant to have fantasy, and the neurobiology of drugs in the ventral tegmental dopaminergic SEEKING system might generate results such as our case series in which 39% of opioid-addicted patients reported dreams of pursuing opioid use, whereas none of the patients who had been maintained on opioid medications as a treatment for chronic pain reported drug dreams.[31]

SUMMARY

1. We make no claim that the engineering models are "true."
2. The models are based on neuroscience combined with clinical experience.
3. Although animal research may contribute to models, the goal is to help humans. Therefore, models are congruent with human experiences.
4. Models improve outcomes for addicted patients including survival, physical and mental health, and function.

The models allow for interlocking concepts that form the backdrop of treatment.

1. Understanding the finances of the addictive drug industry undercuts a common countertransference that addicted patients are lying drug abusers, or that getting high is a hedonistic activity. It is the very opposite. Patients have been using addictive drugs since childhood to cut off horrible emotional signals about having been abused. Calling it *getting high* is best understood as a way to describe the relief of temporary escape from traumatic experiences and memories without having to consciously acknowledge unconscious fantasies that involve "mental representations, those concerned with conflicting wishes, affects, and defensive maneuvers." Addiction is a desperate adaptation to adverse human environments. As treaters we are trying to rescue a few of the victims of an unacknowledged mass killing unparalleled in human history. The methodology involves taking complex human experiences that are responded to behaviorally but not consciously understood and putting them painstakingly into words. Words and conscious representations of feelings, memories and experience counter the impulse to act addictively.
2. Addiction taking over the will informs our treatment approach. Explanations about why addictive drugs are used don't make sense to us. Treatment can be informed by this fact. An interpretation from the treating psychotherapist that their denial is simply reiterating, "I want to use drugs," may help the patient appreciate that this urgent, impelling wish is lodged permanently inside them.
3. Drive and instinct are nicely separated using Panksepp's 7 neural pathways. The SEEKING drive is overarching and will trump hedonic instinctual systems; LUST, CARE, and PLAY, which is why addicted patients neglect their lovers and children while single-mindedly pursuing drugs.
4. From a cultural view, we live in a society that tolerates legal profit making by killing with drugs. Children grow up under extremely adverse conditions and then become the victims of these killers. Awareness of this aspect of mass psychology locates patient and treater in a reality that informs their interaction.

REFERENCES

1. Koh HH. Global tobacco control as a health and human rights imperative. Harvard Int Law J 2016;57:433–53.
2. Lai S, Lai H, Page JB, et al. The association between cigarette smoking and drug abuse in the United States. J Addict Dis 2000;19:11–24.
3. Available at: http://www.idph.state.il.us/public/hb/hbsmoke.htm. Accessed November 20, 2017.
4. Available at: https://www.niaaa.nih.gov/alcohol-health/overview-alcohol-consumption/alcohol-facts-and-statistics. Accessed November 20, 2017.
5. Auchincloss EL. The psychoanalytic model of the mind. Washington, DC: American Psychiatric Publishing; 2015.
6. SAMHSA. National Survey of Drug Use and Health. 2015.
7. National Institute of Health: NIDA, NIAAA websites.
8. Available at: https://www.nytimes.com/interactive/2017/06/05/upshot/opioid-epidemic-drug-overdose-deaths-are-rising-faster-than-ever.html?mcubz=0. Accessed November 20, 2017.
9. Benzodiazepines: $509. Available at: http://www.bendbulletin.com/localstate/2119922-151/benzodiazepines-treat-anxiety-cause-long-term-problems. Accessed November 20, 2017.
10. Alcohol: $212 Alcoholic beverage market overview in the United States. Available at: www.parkstreet.com/alcoholic-beverage-market-overview/. Accessed November 20, 2017.
11. Tobacco: $50. Available at: https://iiwisdom.com/mo-2017/wp-content/uploads/sites/172/2017/04/Altria-Group-Inc.-2016-Annual-Report.pdf. Accessed November 20, 2017.
12. Marijuana, if legalized: $45. Available at: https://taxfoundation.org/marijuana-tax-legalization-federal-revenue/#_ftnref5. Accessed November 20, 2017.
13. Mexican/Columbian Drug Cartels: $29 NYTimes. 2012.
14. Opioid Medications: $19 CNBC on 4/27/16 reported $24 billion/year for opioid medications, 80% sold in the US.
15. Automotive Industry: $70. Available at: https://www.statista.com/topics/1721/us-automotive-industry/. Accessed November 20, 2017.
16. Endy D. Foundations for engineering biology. Nature 2005;438:449–53.
17. Available at: https://en.wikipedia.org/wiki/Systems_engineering. Accessed November 20, 2017.
18. Johnson B, Mosri D. The Neuropsychoanalytic approach: using neuroscience as the basic science of psychoanalysis. Front Psychol 2016;7:1459.
19. Panksepp J. Affective neuroscience. NewYork: Oxford University Press; 1998.
20. Panksepp J, Biven L. The archeology of mind. NewYork: Norton; 2012.
21. Johnson B. Pleasure principle. In: Zeigler-Hill V, Shackelford TK, editors. Encyclopedia of personality and individual differences. Springer International Publishing AG; 2017. https://doi.org/10.1007/978-3-319-28099-8_1411-1.
22. Johnson B. Just what lies beyond the pleasure principle? Neuropsychoanalysis 2008;10:201–12.
23. Goldstein RB, Chou S, Saha TD, et al. The epidemiology of antisocial behavioral syndromes in adulthood: results from the national epidermiologic survey on alcohol and related conditions-III. J Clin Psychiatry 2017;78(1):90–8.
24. Erreich A. Unconscious fantasy as a special class of mental representation: a contribution to a model of mind. J Am Psychoanal Assn 2017;65:195–215, 204.
25. Johnson B. Addiction and will. Front Hum Neurosci 2013;7:545.

26. Nesse RM, Berridge KC. Psychoactive drug use in evolutionary perspective. Science 1997;278:63–6.
27. Hser Y, Evans E, Huang D, et al. Long-term outcomes after randomization to buprenorphine/naloxone versus methadone in a multi-site trial. Addiction 2016;111: 695–705.
28. Johnson B. Psychological addiction, physical addiction, addictive character, addictive personality disorder: a new nosology of addiction. Canadian Journal of Psychoanalysis 2003;11:135–60.
29. Johnson B. Psychoanalytic treatment of psychological addiction to alcohol (alcohol abuse). Front Psychol 2011;2:362.
30. Solms M, Turnbull O. The brain and the inner world: an introduction to the neuroscience of subjective experience. New York: Other Press; 2002.
31. Johnson B, Faraone SV. Outpatient detoxification completion and one month outcomes for opioid dependence: a preliminary open label study of a neuropsychoanalytic treatment in pain patients and addicted patients. Neuropsychoanalysis 2013;15:145–60.